YOU KNOW WHAT YOU WANT—NOW GET IT!

Take control of your own sexual pleasure in seven potent steps. Graham Masterton shares the titillating techniques that real women can use to free their bodies and minds—and make their men respond in ways they never thought possible. It's the ultimate guide to the wildest, hottest, most intense sex of your life!

Discover how to:

- Release your strongest inhibitions
- Seduce your man into acting the way *you* want him to
- Spice up your sex life with both ancient and modern techniques
- Dare to make your wildest fantasies come true
- And more!

THE 7 SECRETS OF REALLY GREAT SEX

Graham Masterton

A SIGNET BOOK

SIGNET
Published by the Penguin Group
Penguin Putnam Inc., 375 Hudson Street,
New York, New York 10014, U.S.A.
Penguin Books Ltd, 27 Wrights Lane,
London W8 5TZ, England
Penguin Books Australia Ltd, Ringwood,
Victoria, Australia
Penguin Books Canada Ltd, 10 Alcorn Avenue,
Toronto, Ontario, Canada M4V 3B2
Penguin Books (N.Z.) Ltd, 182–190 Wairau Road,
Auckland 10, New Zealand

Penguin Books Ltd, Registered Offices:
Harmondsworth, Middlesex, England

First published by Signet, an imprint of Dutton NAL,
a member of Penguin Putnam Inc.

First Printing, March, 1999
10 9 8 7 6 5 4 3 2 1

Printed in the United States of America

Contents

Introduction: Sex—The Good and the Great

In truth, there is only one basic secret of really great sex, although this book will show you seven different ways it can transform your love life.

That secret is for you to take control of your own sexual pleasure. In other words, don't leave your arousal and satisfaction to anybody else, not even to your husband or your lover. Only you know what you really want out of your sex life. Only you can achieve it. If you're looking for guaranteed excitement and guaranteed fulfillment, you'll have to discover for yourself exactly what you want out of your lovemaking and how to make it happen. Once you've done that, you will have the ability to turn humdrum, everyday sex into really good sex, and really good sex into really outstanding sex.

And the more *you* enjoy it, the more your partner will enjoy it, too.

"But excuse me," many women have told me, "we don't *want* to be in control of our love lives. The whole excitement of having sex with a man is that *he* takes control, and that he dominates us. Sometimes it's very arousing to feel helpless, to feel that a man is 'having his way' with us."

Gabby, a 32-year-old teacher from Cedar Rapids, Iowa, said, "There isn't anything more exciting than being pinned down on the bed while a big, muscular man shoves his huge cock into you."

And Sarah, a 27-year-old computer operator from Seattle, Washington, went even further. "My number one sexual fantasy is to have one man's great big hard cock in my pussy, another one up my ass, and a third one right down my throat, all at once. They're all rough and grunting and sweaty. But what turns me on so much is the idea of being *used*. Not very feminist, I know."

Maybe it doesn't *sound* very feminist, but these days you can have it both ways, so to speak. If you enjoy your lover being dominant in bed, there are ways to encourage him to act that way that will ensure that you get all the excitement of being "helpless" while still making sure that he gives you all the stimulation and all the satisfaction to which you're more than entitled.

Theoretically, at least, we now live in a world of sexual equality, and it has long been recognized that a woman's sexual needs are just as great as those of a man. But it's no use ignoring the simple biological truth that women *do* get aroused by men behaving in a sexually assertive way. Maybe not all the time. It depends on the man and it depends upon what kind of relationship you have. But there is no question that it is a fundamental part of what makes a man physically attractive to a woman. Take the enduring appeal of Rhett Butler in *Gone With the Wind,* and all the scenes of forcible sex that you can find in women's popular fiction.

"He pushed her up against the cinderblock wall. 'Jack,' she gasped, as he lifted her skirt up around her waist. 'Not here, Jack. Don't.' But he was far too strong for her. His kisses crushed against her lips, and his unshaven chin scratched against her cheeks. He dragged down her panties and then lifted her up in both hands. She struggled and twisted and pulled at his hair, but when his bone-hard erection forced its way into her, and she slowly sank down onto it, her struggles became shivers of pleasure, and her tugs became caresses. . . ."

We're not talking about allowing your lover to treat you like a sex object. This kind of rough, aggressive coupling may be exciting in books and movies, but in real life it's almost invariably the result of the man's selfishness and sexual ignorance. In real life, *he* usually gets his rocks off, leaving *you* feeling bruised, humiliated, and very dissatisfied.

No, what we're talking about is encouraging your

lover to be active and virile, both for his pleasure and yours. Of course you want him to *believe* that he's completely in charge. That will increase his sense of domination. But to get the optimum pleasure and excitement out of your lovemaking, he will almost certainly need considerable guidance. Men aren't psychic, and when it comes to sex, few of them are very knowledgeable. High school biology lessons and the "Playboy Advisor" may have given your lover a general idea of female sexual anatomy and the notion that women are entitled to orgasms. But you can't expect him to know intuitively what kind of stimulation you enjoy the most, or what kind of sexual scenarios you find the most arousing.

Jane, a 23-year-old beautician from Phoenix, Arizona, told me, "It takes me a long time to get aroused, so I really love it when a man goes down on me and gives me oral sex as part of his foreplay . . . the longer the better. But even though I tried to persuade my last boyfriend to do it, he was always too impatient to get his cock inside me. He licked me there once or twice, but then it was 'Come on, baby, let's do it,' and by the time he'd done it and finished I wasn't even halfway there." Failure to kiss and arouse them properly is the number one complaint leveled by women against their husbands and lovers by *far*.

Then there's a lack of spontaneity. Rachel, a 26-year-old airline steward from Cincinnati, Ohio, said, "I love to have sex outdoors. In the woods, in the fields. I love running around naked and feeling the breeze on my skin when I'm making love. But when I took my last boyfriend out to the lake and said, 'Doesn't this make you feel romantic? Doesn't this make you feel like making love?' all he could say was 'It sure does. . . . I can't wait to get you back home.' Don't get me wrong. He was a very red-blooded guy. But he didn't see how excited I was by the idea of having sex in the open. In the end, the only way I could get him to make love to me was to open up his pants, take out his cock, and give him a long, slow blow job. I thought it was great. The sun was shining on his cock and it was bright red and glistening with saliva. But even then he was very uneasy, you know? He didn't feel comfortable at all. Maybe he was worried that somebody might be watching, but that never worries me. In fact that's part of the buzz. Let's just say that he didn't exactly behave like Tarzan."

When it comes to sex, men need very clear signals. There are very few times when your sexual messages can be too obvious. One girl told me that after an evening with a man she really liked, she became so impatient for him to make a move that she took off all her clothes and got into bed. He hesitated for a moment and then he said, "Do you want me to go now?"

Men also need a constant *feedback.* They need to be reassured that they're doing the right thing, and that you're enjoying what they're doing to you—or, if you're *not* enjoying it, they need to know that, too. I have talked to literally hundreds of men over the years, and the women that they have considered to be the sexiest haven't necessarily been the prettiest, or the most flirtatious, or the ones with the biggest breasts. It's the women who have clearly *responded* to their lovemaking—letting them know when a touch has thrilled them, letting them know when a thrust is satisfyingly deep and, conversely, letting them know when they haven't quite been stimulating the right spot, or if they've been handling them too roughly.

In a word, they're looking for women who can give them sexual confidence—women who have enough sexual skill to be able to control the course of their own erotic relationships. Although, of course, they will rarely admit it—sometimes, not even to themselves.

Striking the right balance between over-responsiveness and under-responsiveness can be difficult. Here's Mara, a 26-year-old grade-school teacher from Baltimore, Maryland. "I was brought up in a very puritanical family. My mother never discussed sex or boys. I had quite a thorough sex education at school, but what they don't tell you at school is how to behave when you go to bed with a man. I mean, should you be cool and aloof? Or should you be wildly enthusiastic? I found out about oral sex by talking to my friends but I didn't know what the etiquette was. Can you just put your head down and start sucking a man's cock, or should you have some conversation and a few kisses first? Should you show him how much you're enjoying it? Should you say anything while you're making love or should you stay silent?

"I know it sounds pathetic but I just didn't *know* these things. But I'd seen a couple of movies where the woman goes crazy when she's making love. You know—screaming out 'Harder! Harder!' and digging her nails into the man's back. So when I first went to bed with a man I tried to be all passionate, panting and moaning and wriggling. It was all an act, and it was *so* embarrassing. He said, 'Do you mind shutting up? I can't hear myself fuck.' That was exactly what he said. So when I first went to bed with Richard I was just the opposite. I didn't say a word and I just lay there and said nothing in case it upset him. At the same time, you know, I had no idea what you should allow your lover to do to you and what you shouldn't.

"I think Richard liked it at first because I allowed him to do anything and I never complained. I thought that if I complained that would be the end of our relationship. For instance he used to put his hand up my skirt whenever he felt like it, and finger me. Sometimes he put his hand inside my panties when I was in the kitchen making supper. He used to rub my clitoris and push two or three fingers up inside my pussy. Sometimes he tried to push his whole hand up me and I hated that. But once he fucked me when I was standing over the sink trying to wash lettuce, and that was really sexy.

"He always excited me, but he never seemed to think that I had needs, too. He was always finished before I was, so I was left almost every time with this feeling of frustration. One of his favorite things was to rub his cock between my breasts until he came. I liked that, too, the way he massaged my breasts and my nipples and squeezed them together. I liked it when his sperm shot out all over my face and all over my hair. I can't say that it didn't turn me on, because it did, and I loved to lick it up. But after he had climaxed, that was it. Finished. He climbed off me and went to sleep and if *I* wanted a climax I had to wait until he was asleep and masturbate.

"We still loved each other but everything was falling apart. I was allowing him to treat me like a piece of meat and I felt ashamed of what I was doing, but I was scared of losing him and I didn't know how to assert myself. I never complained. It just goes to show you what an impression your first two or three lovers can have on you. If you're lucky you'll find yourself partners who are experienced and understanding and good in bed, and so you have a way of judging every man you make love to after that. But if your first lovers are clumsy and selfish . . . I mean, how are you supposed to *know* that sex can be a whole lot better?

"With Richard it got to the point where there was

hardly any communication at all, not about sex, and it began to affect the rest of our relationship, too. Sometimes I used to get very irritable and moody and other times I used to burst into tears for no reason. It was my fault as much as his. He didn't know how I felt and I didn't know how to tell him. Even though we were still having sex, we were like two strangers.

"One night I was awakened about three in the morning by this really strange cold feeling between my legs. Richard was smearing almost a whole tube of KY between the cheeks of my ass. The next thing I knew he was trying to push his cock up my butt. I couldn't believe it. I mean, I knew about anal sex but I didn't know that ordinary people did it, people like us. And this was when I was *asleep,* right? No foreplay, nothing. He was just using me.

"It hurt a lot. I mean to begin with I had tears in my eyes. But I stayed perfectly still while he pushed it up farther and farther. I don't know how he did it, because he's enormous when he's hard, but he pushed it all the way up inside me until I could feel his hair up against the cheeks of my ass. I felt like I wanted to squeeze it out of me, but at the same time I felt like I wanted it even deeper inside me. It did excite me. I suppose he knew that it excited me, because he was fingering my pussy at the same time and my pussy was so juicy that I thought that I must have wet myself. But I didn't know how to respond, that was the trouble. I didn't want to scream, although I felt like screaming. I didn't want to wriggle, although I felt like wriggling, with that huge cock buried inside my ass. I guess I was afraid that he would get upset.

"He fucked me very slowly. It seemed to last forever. It didn't stop hurting but it didn't stop feeling good, either. In the end he gave a grunting noise and I could feel his cock bulging when he came. After it was over he held me close but I still didn't say a word. My butt was sore but I was very aroused. I was dying for him to do something else to me, masturbate me or go down on me or *something*, but that was it. The next thing I knew he was fast asleep. I lay there with sperm slowly dripping out of my sore, wide-open asshole, feeling very sorry for myself.

"A couple of days later—totally by surprise—he said that he was going to visit his sister in Silver Spring. He said that things weren't working out between us and he needed to think. I asked him what was wrong. I mean I knew what was wrong from my point of view, but I couldn't understand what was wrong from *his*. We were the best of friends. Sexually, he could do anything he wanted. But he said I was frigid. He said that no matter how hard he tried, he couldn't turn me on. He said I just lay there, and didn't say anything. He said he had fucked me up my ass, which was something he had never done before and always wanted to try, and what had I done? Nothing at all. I hadn't said that I loved it. I hadn't even said that I hated it.

"We had an argument, and he left. But it was then that I began to understand that I had to be myself when it came to sex. I had to stop worrying about Richard and think about *me.* I had to discover what *I* liked and what *I* needed. Then I had to learn how to show Richard what these things were, and how to do them to me. I wasn't a Stepford wife. I wasn't an inflatable doll. I was a real woman with real feelings, and that was what Richard was looking for. That's what *all* men are looking for, if you ask me."

Mara's self-discovery was the turning point in her relationship with Richard, and with all the men she subsequently dated. She realized that she had to take control of what was happening in her sex life, right from the very beginning. Not in the sense of being a control freak, but by making love to her own agenda, and making sure that she was never left dissatisfied. She used some of my earlier books to learn about her own body and her own responses. But most important of all, she learned how to communicate her sexual needs and how to respond when they were met.

A man could be a very experienced and sensitive lover, but that doesn't mean he's psychic. He may know that if he licks your clitoris lightly and quickly, he'll give you the kind of sensation that dreams are made of. But what he won't know, and *can't* know, is that if he licked just a quarter inch lower, and just a little more lightly . . .

You will have to learn how to communicate with

him on many different levels, from lucid and detailed explanations of what your erotic fantasies are, to nudges and winks and kisses and the most suggestive of body language. You will have to learn how to show him what you're feeling without making him think that you're belittling his sexual performance. If you murmur, "Lower . . . a little lower down, that's wonderful. . . ." you won't destroy his ego, or make him feel as if he's some kind of sexual incompetent. Neither will giving a soft moan and moving your hips so that he *has* to lick you lower down. In fact he'll probably be more than glad to know that he's giving you the kind of cunnilingus that's certain to bring you to a satisfying orgasm. You have to involve him in giving you really great sex.

A lack of communication on any level can cause a sexual relationship to break down as quickly and completely as an automobile without oil. Debbie, 36, a sales manager from Dallas, Texas, had a seven-month relationship with Brad, who was four years her junior. "I don't entirely take the blame for what happened, but when I look back on it I guess at least half of it was my fault. I first met Brad at a corporate reception, and I was *instantly* attracted to him. He's tall, six two, with dark curly hair and a very athletic build, like he works out a lot. Right from the beginning he was very polite, very quiet. It was me who suggested that we go for a drink together after the reception, and then on to dinner.

"He was gorgeous. He still *is* gorgeous. But it was

me who asked him back to my apartment for a nightcap, and I suppose it was me who started to kiss him. I took him into the bedroom and undressed him, and let me tell you that he has a body to die for. Muscles, suntan, and hair on his chest, and the biggest cock you ever saw.

"I didn't even take off my high-heeled shoes. I lay back on the bed and lifted up my dress and underneath I was wearing a white lacy garter belt and white stockings and no panties, because I hardly ever wear them. Brad climbed on top of me and I took hold of his cock and guided it between my legs. It was immense, his cock, and incredibly hard. I'll never forget how purple and fat it was, like some kind of ripe juicy fruit that you could sink your teeth into. When it slid inside me, I felt that it was never going to stop. He made love real slow, which was beautiful, and I could feel his big heavy balls banging against me every time he pushed inside. I was in heaven for a while, I really was.

"Then—just when I was beginning to feel that this was going to be the best fuck that I'd ever had in my life—he suddenly took his cock out of me, and gave it two or three rubs, and came all over my stomach. I was splattered all over with warm wet sperm, it seemed like gallons of it, but I was only halfway to having an orgasm. He gave me one kiss, stood up, and went to the bathroom. I tried to bring myself off. I thought *What—is that it?* I was so frustrated that I was panting out loud. I smeared his sperm between my legs and rubbed my clitoris like crazy. But all of that initial excitement had gone, and before I was even halfway there he came back from the bathroom with this self-satisfied look on his face, and I had to stop.

"I thought he was so good looking, and I still do. I mean, he's an *Adonis.* He asked me out to dinner that weekend; of course I went. This time we went back to his place and we made love again, but it was just the same. He got me all excited, and then wham, bam, out came his cock, all over my thighs, all over the sheets, and that was the finish. The trouble was I didn't know how to tell him without upsetting him. But it seemed to me that his only sexual experiences must have been with very young girls who hadn't been able to show him what a real woman wanted.

"I guess I could have shown him myself. I *should* have shown him. But I admit that I didn't want to take the risk of losing him. He could have any woman he wanted, but I wanted that woman to be me. But of course things didn't get any better.

"After six weeks, though, his lovemaking really began to get on my nerves. I tried to tell him about it one time, but as soon as I said, 'Listen . . . about the way you make love . . .' he said, 'Really . . . you don't have to pay me any compliments.' And I didn't want to push it any further because I got the feeling that he'd take it real hard.

"I talked to my girlfriends, and they said, 'What are you complaining about, we'd do anything to have a young stud jerking himself off all over us.' But he frustrated me, he *bored* me, if you must know, and yet he still seemed to think that he was the greatest stud on God's good earth. I tried to say things like 'I'd love to feel you coming inside of me,' but either he didn't understand or else he was so fixed in his ways that he couldn't come any other way.

"We had more and more spats, and in the end we agreed not to see each other for a while, which turned into a *very* long while. As I say, I still think he's gorgeous, but I should have found a way of showing him where he was going wrong. Or rather, where he was *coming* wrong."

Personally, I think that Debbie was being much too hard on herself. I'm always amazed how many women take the blame for dysfunctional sexual relationships when it is obvious that the cause of the problem is their partner's ignorance, selfishness, clumsiness, or all three. The wife of a TV soap star appeared on television with a black eye and blamed herself for provoking her partner into hitting her, as well as for his extramarital affair.

The way to sort out a sexual problem in your relationship is not to take the blame, but to take control. It was obvious, for instance, that Brad was virile but utterly self-centered. For most women, feeling her lover ejaculate inside her, knowing that he *wants* to ejaculate inside her, is part of the emotional and biological fulfillment of intercourse. But occasionally one encounters men like Brad who insist, on every occasion, on taking out their penises prior to their climax and watching themselves ejaculate. It could have been vanity—admiring his own sperm shooting out. It could have been a way of humiliating her. Many men derive sexual excitement from ejaculating in women's faces and over their bodies. It's also possible that he learned all of his sexual technique from porn videos, where a visible "come shot" is mandatory.

But I think that Debbie herself was closest to the truth when she said that maybe he couldn't come any other way. Taking out his penis and masturbating himself to a climax had become a ritual—a fetish, almost—and it would take a great deal of patient guidance to help him overcome it.

Given that she was prepared to *be* patient, there were many ways in which Debbie could have taken control of their sexual relationship, to change Brad's behavior and turn him into the kind of lover that she really wanted. Brad needn't even have been aware of the changes that she was making—just as you can change your lover without him ever being aware of it (unless you leave this book lying on his pillow).

One of the simplest techniques she could have used was to roll him over halfway through lovemaking so that she was sitting astride him. Even if she were quite slim, her weight would have been enough to prevent him from taking out his penis when he came close to his climax—particularly if she made sure that she sat upright. If she were on her back and found it physically impossible to roll him over and sit on top of him, then she could simply have put her hands down between his legs and clutched his testicles. If she felt that he was close to a climax, and preparing to pull himself out, she could have dug in her fingernails, if necessary, for extra excitement, but also for extra control.

If she were still physically unable to prevent him from taking out his penis, another way in which she could have weaned him off the habit of openly ejaculating would have been to go down on him as soon as he took it out and give him oral sex—completely swallowing his sperm when he climaxed so that he didn't get to see it. Whether she would have been prepared to do that or not would have been up to her own personal taste. Some women dislike swallowing their lover's sperm, but I have come across many more who say that they can't get enough of it. The important psychological principle, though, was that Debbie should have made sure that Brad became accustomed to ejaculating inside her, as the climax of their sexual togetherness, instead of making a sideshow out of it.

Once she had succeeded in having him ejaculate inside her, she should then have lavished him with praise. "That was wonderful . . . you've filled me right up. I didn't think I could take that much sperm inside me." Unless he was Neanderthal man, he would then be likely to get the message that she was pleased and excited by what he had done, and be more inclined to repeat the performance the next time they made love. There would be no obvious indication that she had contrived what had happened, or that it had been the result of anything else but his own virility.

Learning to take control of your sexual relationships calls for a whole lot of tact, even more determination, and a strong belief in your own sexiness. Maybe your partner hasn't appreciated up until now just how sexy you are. Maybe you've been together for so long that he simply takes you for granted. Either way, you're going to make him stiffen up and take notice, and give you all the sexual treats you've ever imagined.

You need to build up your own sexual confidence so that you are quite sure of your own physical attractiveness and your own skill as your lover's lover. So many women are still cheating themselves of really great sex because they don't believe that they're particularly alluring, and they can't convince themselves that they're any good in bed.

But no matter what you think about your physical appearance . . . whether you think you're overweight or underweight . . . whether you don't like your nose or your hair or the size of your breasts . . . you have the potential to be the sexiest woman that the man in your life ever met. Later in this book I'll show you how.

Next, you need to face up to all of your sexual anxieties and all of your sexual inhibitions. Is there anything about your sex life that worries you? Do you know what happens to your body when you're sexually excited? Do you know what happens when your lover becomes sexually excited (apart from the obvious)? Are you confident that you know what arouses your lover the most—and, if you do know, are you prepared to do it? What do you feel about oral sex? And did you know that over 85 percent of men counted oral sex as their favorite sexual variation?

Are there any sexual acts that you think you could never, ever think of performing—such as anal sex or wet sex or bondage—but that you suspect that your lover might want to try?

If you're in control of your love life, there are plenty of ways of diverting his attention to other sexual practices that will give him just as much of a thrill. But this book will show you how you can overcome your inhibitions if you want to, and learn to enjoy some of the most extreme sexual acts imaginable.

Anthea, 31, a dancer from Anaheim, California, said, "When I was younger, the very *idea* of anal sex used to make me feel goosebumpy. I couldn't believe that people actually did it. But I read one of your books about how to prepare yourself for anal sex, and I was living alone then, and I tried it. Now I can't get enough of it. I love it. And I'm proud to say that one night, after a party, I managed to get two men up my asshole both at once, one black and one white, and they weren't under-endowed, either! It was a struggle, but it was amazing!"

From St. Petersburg, Florida, 36-year-old Rhoda, a

homemaker, wrote, "I read your latest book and I was very turned on by your descriptions of wet sex, which is something that has always secretly excited me but which I have never dared to mention to any of my partners. Two nights ago, however, I invited my husband, Mel, into the bathroom where I was sitting on the john. I was wearing nothing but white lace panties. I said, 'Watch this,' and I pissed without taking my panties off. Then I opened up his jeans and said, 'It's your turn, you can make my panties wet, too.' He was so hard that he could hardly piss, but in the end he managed it. He pissed between my legs and I slid my hand into my panties and rubbed myself while he was doing it. Then he pissed all over my breasts and down my stomach. We finished up on the bathroom floor doing sixty-nine . . . me sucking his piss-flavored cock and him pulling aside my panties and licking my soaking cunt. Then I climbed on top of him and it was the most exciting sex I'd ever had. You made me feel that I could do anything without feeling guilty or dirty or ashamed, and you don't know how much you've liberated me, especially as a woman, since pissing for women is always so 'private.' Now I like to do it in the shower, standing up, before I turn on the water. I splash it all over my breasts and masturbate myself and I love every minute of it."

Ricky, 24, an assistant for a large realty corporation in Orlando, Florida, said, "My boyfriend, Rex, was always talking about bondage and that movie with

Sharon Stone in it—what was it?—*Basic Instinct.* I never liked the idea of bondage. It frightened me. But then I read in one of your books that bondage could be exciting so long as you stuck to certain rules, and I guess that was what convinced me to try it . . . although I did tell Rex that he had to keep to the rules like *religiously* or else it was all going to be over between us. One evening he filled the bedroom with scented candles and then he undressed me and tied my wrists and ankles to the bed. He used silk scarves. They're soft, but they tighten pretty quick if you try to struggle. He blindfolded me, too, so that I couldn't see anything at all. He put on some really soft, weird music that kind of disoriented me, you know? Then he began to kiss me and touch me all over and there was nothing I could do to stop him. He played with my breasts and sucked my nipples. Then he slowly kissed me and licked me all over, and I mean all over.

"It's kind of scary at first, being completely helpless like that, but once you relax it's amazing. And you're not really helpless, because when you like something that he's doing to you, you can moan and move your hips and show him that he's really turning you on.

"He kissed me on the lips and then he brushed his stiff cock against my lips. I kept sticking my tongue out, trying to lick it, but he teased me by taking it just out of reach. Then, without any warning at all, he pushed it right into my mouth. I started to suck it, but he took it out again. He rubbed it against my nipples and between my breasts and then he slid it down my stomach and rubbed it against my bellybutton.

"He went on teasing me and teasing me. He kissed me all around my cunt and then he kissed the inside of my thighs all the way down to my knees. He licked and sucked my toes. Then he went back to kissing my cunt again, and this time he slid his tongue inside me and then he started licking my clitoris, so lightly that it was like having a butterfly beating its wings between my legs.

"Just when I felt that I was rising toward an orgasm, he stopped licking my clitoris and kissed my breasts again. It felt wonderful, but the frustration was almost too much, and because I was tied up there was nothing that I could do about it!

"I said, 'Fuck me, please fuck me,' but he wouldn't, and when I kept on saying it again and again he pushed his cock back into my mouth and said 'Ssh!' to stop me from saying it again. I didn't mind that. I was so turned on by then that I could have swallowed it all the way down, but then he took it out and rolled it against my breasts again. I wanted him to fuck me so much I was almost screaming.

"In the end he ran his tongue around my thighs and licked between the cheeks of my ass. Then he started to lick my clitoris in earnest, not too hard, not too fast, but on and on and on, taking me up, do you know what I mean? Taking me up. I felt my orgasm coming. I felt it coming like a big dark train, bell ringing, whistle blowing. Because there I was, all tied up, with my legs wide apart, and no matter what Rex wanted to do to me, I couldn't do anything about it. I just prayed that Rex wouldn't stop before I came. But he didn't, he kept on licking me, and even when my orgasm went through me and I was jumping and jerking around on the bed and screaming at the top of my voice, he *still* went on licking me until I couldn't stand it any longer and I had to *beg* him to stop.

"But it was then that he climbed on top of me and pushed his cock inside me. My cunt was still rippling, and he made me come again and again—you know, like aftershocks. He fucked me very, very slowly, and every now and then he took his cock out of me and rubbed the head of it around the lips of my cunt, and up against my clitoris, until I was beginning to feel that another orgasm was on the way, a really big one. I was tied up, so there was hardly anything I could do. I couldn't touch him, I couldn't kiss him, I couldn't rub him. But I squeezed my cunt muscles as tight as I could, trying to grip his cock each time that it was deep inside me. He must have felt it almost at once, because he pushed himself right up inside me as far as he could go, and just lay there on top of me, while I squeezed his cock in this really sexy rhythm, you know, like a bossa nova. Only you wouldn't have known that we were doing it, if you'd walked into the room and seen us. It was all inside of us, you know? Inside our bodies.

"When I came for the second time, I wanted to hold him tight, but of course I couldn't. I had never had an orgasm like that before, ever. It shook up my whole soul, believe me. It was like the world exploding inside of my body, and because I couldn't move it seemed to shake me all the more. I couldn't even squeeze my thighs together, which I normally do when I climax. And I felt so open and naked and exposed, like Rex was actually looking at my cunt while I had an orgasm.

"We've tried bondage twice since then, but I'm not sure we're ever going to repeat the experience—not yet, anyway. That first time as so earth-shattering that I think I'd be disappointed if we did it too often. The second time was pretty good, though. I tied Rex to one of the kitchen chairs, with cord. Totally naked, with a blindfold, and a gag in his mouth. I think he was scared, to tell you the truth. I knelt down in front of him, sucked him until he was really hard. Then I sat on his lap, and rode him up and down the way I like it—very, very slowly.

"That's what I *will* say in favor of bondage. You can tease and you can tantalize and your partner can't do anything about it. When Rex was sitting on that chair, I could lift myself up so that his cock was only just inside me, my cunt lips barely clinging to him. Then I could hold myself there for as long as I liked, saying, 'You want to push it right up inside me, don't you? Well, you can't.' And he was gagged, so he couldn't even answer me, even though I knew that he was aching to push himself right up into me. I teased him for almost half an hour. But in the end I rode him so hard and so fast that he couldn't stop himself from coming and I think he would have yelled out if he'd been able to. His come was flying everywhere, and I was so sweaty and exhausted that I practically fell off the chair and lay on my back on the floor. But I didn't untie him until I'd gotten my breath back, and enjoyed the luxury of sucking his cock while it was soft, which is something that he doesn't normally like me to do. Male pride, I guess."

Sexual experimentation can open up all kinds of exciting and arousing experiences. But if you're naturally reserved about sex, or you simply don't feel the need to experiment, you can have a really great love life without doing anything extreme or unusual. In some of the most intense and long-lasting sexual relationships that I have ever seen, the couples have almost only ever made love in completely conventional ways. By that I mean straightforward intercourse—no acrobatic positions, no fantasy role-playing, no handcuffs.

That's because the basis of really great sex is knowing how to please your lover both physically and mentally—no matter how you do it—and how to teach him to do the same to you. It's knowing how to open up your body and your mind, and getting him to open up *his* body and *his* mind. It's sharing the intensity of your pleasure. The basis of really great sex is becoming one, if only for an instant.

So, provided you and your lover both feel that you're enjoying all of the sexual excitement that you possibly can, provided neither of you have the feeling that you're missing out on something, it doesn't matter if you stick to the "missionary position" for the rest of your relationship.

You should, however, keep an open mind about sexual variations, because once you've overcome any initial reservations that you might have about them, many of them can be exciting and fun.

Incidentally, don't mistake a sexual *variation* for a sexual *fetish,* which is something completely different. You might give your lover an occasional thrill by dressing up in rubber, but if it is critical to his sexual satisfaction that you're dressed from head to toe in latex, then he has a clinical condition. This applies to any variation, such as spanking or shoe fetishism or cross-dressing. You may feel—as many women do—that their lover's fetish isn't a problem. For instance, many wives have very successful relationships with husbands who have a need to dress in women's clothing, and even help them to choose what to wear. One wife from St. Paul, Minnesota, told me that her husband liked to dress as a maid on weekends, naked except for a frilly apron and high stiletto heels. He cooked all the meals and cleaned the house until it sparkled, and she certainly had no complaints, especially since their lovemaking afterward was always "fantastic." Sexual fetishes may appear disturbing, but with some exceptions, such as extreme masochistic or sadistic practices, they're pretty harmless.

If you and your lover experiment with sexual variations there's no risk of you turning into deviants overnight. Like Rita, you may find that a few experiences of bondage or cross-dressing or exhibitionism are enough to enliven your love life without having to buy into a lifetime of unusual sex. It shakes you out of your routine. It can help you to look at each other afresh, and remember what it is that excited you about each other in the first place.

My experience as sex counselor over the past twenty-five years has shown me not only how important communication can be, but how critical constantly updated sexual communication is. Like every other intense experience, sex with the same person becomes familiar and loses its capacity to thrill. Any collector of porn videos will tell you how quickly the excitement of a new release starts to pall, and it has been noticeable over the years that titles are becoming more and more extreme in order to titillate a viewing audience that has seen it all.

I have a catalog that shows a Danish sex movie from the early 1970s with two blonde girls in a simulated lesbian scene. It was considered daring at the time because they were shaved. A more recent catalog offers: "A very pretty girl attempting to blow three stiff cocks at once! Soon all three monster pricks empty their loads on her lips and mouth as she greedily swallows every drop. Lots of anal, beautiful girls and a particularly pretty colored chick. Fantastic slow-speed cum shots." And that's one of the milder videos offered.

Even in a comparatively short-term sexual relationship, you can keep up the intensity by constantly coming up with little sexual surprises. In a longer-term relationship, you should make a special point of ensuring that your lovemaking is as fresh and stimulating as it ever was. When two people live together, each can grow to assume that their partner magically knows what they're thinking about, what their desires are, what they're frustrated about. But although a certain degree of "telepathy" can develop between a couple in a long-term sexual relationship, more often than not they grow out of the habit of spelling out to each other the fact that they love each other, and they forget to communicate their feelings about their lovemaking.

After only a few years, many lovers have sex on a routine basis only. They no longer experiment. They no longer feel it necessary to reach for the outer limits of sexual experience. And even if they still harbor sexual fantasies, they no longer have the courage to tell their partners what they are. They've settled down, not wanting to risk the everyday comfort of their existence by telling their partner that they've always had a hankering to make a sex video of the two of them making love, and play it back while they're making love yet again. Or that they'd like to make love in the backyard, at night. Or that they'd like to try a vibrator.

Too many lovers have sexual fantasies that they would like to act out, but are too embarrassed to admit to. Yes, you—and your partner, too. One of the greatest achievements in developing a really great sex life is for each of you to discover your most arousing sexual fantasies and give yourselves the opportunity to bring them to life. Even if they turn out to be too extreme for you to want to try them for real, you can at least describe them and discuss them, and use your discussion as part of your foreplay.

Again, we're talking about communication. Not just physical communication, but the sharing of dreams and intimate desires. If you don't know what your lover secretly wants, then you can't possibly encourage him to bring his fantasies to life.

Here are six women who persuaded their partners to tell them what their secret sexual fantasies were, and their reactions. Georgina, 33, from St. Louis, Missouri: "After a few drinks, Greg finally managed to tell me that he'd always wanted me to go out with him wearing no panties. Nobody else would know, only him; and I would give him glimpses of my naked cunt whenever I could—climbing in and out of the car, bending over to pick up a package, sitting cross-legged on a couch. My cunt hair is bright red, just like the hair on my head, and he's always said how much it excites him, but I never knew how much. I was shocked when he first said it, but I think it's a pretty sexy idea, and I think it might turn me on, too. I'll try it one day, but I won't tell him first. It'll be a surprise."

Jennifer, 26, from Oakland, California: "We swapped fantasies. I told Ray that I had always wanted to dress him up in black stockings before he made love to me. That blew his mind, I can tell you! But then he said that he had always fantasized about me spending the whole day in the nude, even when he was dressed, so that he could touch me and make love to me whenever he felt like it. In a way, I found that a very disturbing fantasy, like he was trying to make me into some kind of sexual plaything, you know? Or like a slave. But in another way I found it very flattering. I don't know. I may try it for real. I think I may find it quite sexy to be totally naked all day, even when I'm cooking supper!"

Renata, 25, from New York, New York: "We were having a discussion late at night and Jake asked me if there was one physical thing that I would change about him, what was it? And I said his front teeth, that's all, because they're crooked and it makes him shy about smiling. And so I said, 'What would you change about me?' And he said, 'Nothing, nothing at all, although there is something.' So I said, 'What? My nose, what?' And he said no, he'd like me to shave off all of my pubic hair, so that my pussy was completely bare. And I said, 'You'd really like that?' And he said, 'That would be the greatest turn-on ever.' And we started talking about something else.

But that night, when I climbed into bed, I took his hand and guided it down between my legs . . . and guess what? Smooth, bare pussy, no hair at all. And he had the biggest hard-on in history."

Margarita, 19, from San Diego, California: "Whenever we made love, Carlos was always touching my asshole—you know, trying to push his finger up it, and I said, 'You know, don't keep doing that. Sometimes I like it and sometimes I don't.' So he said that what he really wanted to do was make love to my asshole properly. I said no, I didn't think I wanted to. But what I was really thinking was, how can I possibly fit that huge cock up inside a tiny hole like that? But I read in your book about practicing with vibrators, and I love Carlos, so I practiced, first with a small one and then with a bigger one. Then after three months I said to him one night, 'Come on, Carlos, you can try it.' He didn't know what I meant until I turned around and guided his cock toward my asshole. Then he was in seventh heaven, and to my surprise, so was I."

Jane, 22, from Spokane, Washington: "I didn't know anything at all about bondage until I moved in with Rod. Then one day I was tidying his shorts and his socks when I found this thing that looked like a muzzle for a very small dog—you know, it was kind of black leather and studs and with a metal ring attached. I asked Rod what it was and he was embarrassed at first and didn't want to tell me. But in the end he said it was a cock ring. I asked him to show me how it worked and he really didn't want to, but I'm a very persuasive lady! He slid the ring around the base of his cock and fastened the leather strap tight around his balls, so that they bulged right out. His cock rose up enormously stiff—so stiff that the metal ring was much too tight for it. He said that was the point of it—the only way to get the ring off now would be to have a climax. I didn't say a word. I pulled my skirt up to my waist and pulled my panties to one side and I sat down on that big hard cock until I could feel the metal ring. It was incredible. There was this feeling that we were doing something kinky, and I'd never felt him so big! It seemed to take him much longer to come, too. I could feel his cock swelling and swelling and it was so hard inside me it was like a bone. When he did come, he held me tight and he shouted out loud and he seemed to go on pumping out sperm forever. Afterward I asked him if he was really into this kind of stuff, you know, bondage and leather. He said it turned him on, that's all. He didn't know why. He didn't want me to think that he was a pervert or anything like that. I thought it was great. A little bit kinky, you know, and *very* exciting. So I persuaded him to buy some more things. Now he has a leather harness that I can lace his cock up into, very tight, and a ring that goes around his cock with a strap that divides his balls. It has a clip on it so I can chain him up! We don't use them very often. Most of the time we have a perfectly normal sex life like everybody else. But we have a lot of fun with them when we do. I even made Rod wear his cock ring to my office party, under his pants. He spent the whole evening trying to hide his hard-on!

"I think I might be worried if Rod wanted to wear bondage stuff every time we made love. But as it is, I think it's fun, and if we both enjoy it, where's the harm? Apart from that, I think I'd rather *know* about it than have Rod keep it a secret."

Jane's right, of course. Even if she didn't want to participate in Rod's (very mild) bondage fantasy, she could talk about it with him, and excite him during lovemaking by describing how she would like to strap him and bind him and restrain him.

Phillipa, 29, from Charleston, South Carolina: "We'd been together for about four months when Grant first mentioned the time that he was caught having sex with a girl in a parking lot. He told it as if it was a funny story, but the way he said it, I could tell that it must have given him quite a buzz because after that first time he talked about it again and again. In the end I said, 'Why don't you and me have sex in a parking lot, then you can forget about *her* and what a big thrill she was, and you can start thinking about me instead.' He just laughed and told me to forget about it. But a week later, when we went to the mall, I waited until we were parked and then I said, 'Look,' and I lifted up my dress so that he could see that I was completely naked underneath. To cut the story short, we had sex in the parking lot, and even though we didn't get caught, Grant was so excited about it that I think it took all of his self-control not to call up all of his friends and tell them how great it was. As far as he was concerned, what put the frosting on the cake was when we were walking around the market and I said, 'Do you have a tissue?' and he said 'Why?' and I said, 'Because your come is sliding down my leg.' I think he would have made love to me again, right there and then, in the middle of the vegetable display, if he'd had the strength."

All of the women in these examples improved their sex lives because they were prepared to listen to what their lovers wanted, and within reasonable limits, to give it to them. At the same time they made sure that their own needs were satisfied, too.

It isn't always easy to discover what secret sexual fantasies your husband or your lover may have. Some men have very bizarre fantasies that they are reluctant to describe to their partners for fear of disgusting them. Some women do, too! In many cases they have no real need or desire to act these fantasies out for real, and they only think about them when they are sexually aroused.

But if you can find out what your lover's fantasies are, you will be in a much better position to give him really great sex. First of all, though, you should make sure that you are in a sexually receptive frame of mind. This will enable you to pick up on those clues that will tell you if there is something extra that your lover would like to be doing in bed (or even in the market), and what it is.

Being in a sexually receptive frame of mind will also make you less shockable. I can't count the number of times that women have said to me, "I asked him what he fantasized about, and when he told me, I couldn't believe it—it was so *filthy*!" If you want really great sex, you will have to be knowledgeable, non-judgmental, and very open-minded. And keep remembering that a fantasy is only a fantasy.

So let's explore the first of the seven secrets of really great sex . . . for every women who has pleasure on her mind.

Secret 1: Think Sexy

"I never thought of myself as being sexy. Not in the sense of being the kind of woman who turns heads whenever she walks into a roomful of men. And not in the sense of being adventurous in bed. I'm not saying that I never think about sex. Of course I do, and I love making love. But it always seemed to me that it was other women who did all the flirting, and other women who did all those outrageous things that you read about in the magazines."

This was Patricia, 35, a geriatric nurse from San Diego, California. Patricia was single, although she had just finished, "by mutual consent," an eight-year relationship with an aeronautical engineer named Don. Well, she said the break-up was by mutual consent, but I sensed that she was harboring a deep sense of loss and that she had suffered a severe blow to her sexual confidence.

In contrast, here's Caroline, 21, a liberal arts student from Tallahassee, Florida. "I was never the sexy one. Whenever a group of us girls went out, I was always the one who never got a boy. I could never work out why. I was never overweight, I was always well dressed. I think I was just as pretty as most of my friends. But it just never happened. Well, hardly ever. And when I did get boys they just used to sit there fidgeting and looking at their watches as if they couldn't wait for the date to be over.

"When I graduated from high school and went to college I decided that this was going to change. *I* was going to be the girl who got all the boys. And I did. The second night I was there I invited this boy called Dean back to my room and we drank wine and I opened up his jeans and I practically raped him. The next week I went out with one of the guys from the football team and he was tremendous—physically, anyway. He had these narrow hips and this stomach like rock and a cock that never seemed to go down.

"Everything was fantastic for the first month or so. I must have slept with eleven or twelve guys. I felt sexy, I felt wanted. I felt like the most desirable woman in the whole world. One night I had two boys in my bed at once, and we had sex practically all night, over and over. The things we did! I was so sore the next morning I couldn't wear jeans.

"But none of the guys I went with ever seemed to

want a lasting relationship. Most of the other girls had steady beaux, but after we'd had sex, my guys started looking at their watches all over again. Then they started making excuses why they couldn't go out with me. And it didn't help that hardly any of the girls would speak to me, either. I realized that I wasn't the most desirable woman in the whole world. I was just the same old me with a bad reputation. I guess that was the first time I really understood that good sex isn't just in the body; it has to be there in your mind."

Both Patricia and Caroline wanted sex and enjoyed sex when they had it. But they both lacked real faith in their own sexuality, and before any woman can have really great sex she has to *think* sexy as well as *act* sexy. It's like learning a foreign language. You may know all the vocabulary and all of the grammar, but until you can actually *think* in that language, you won't be able to enjoy a spontaneous conversation.

So no matter how much you know about sex and sexual variations, no matter how much you know about men and how to give them all the pleasure they're looking for, you won't be able to take full control of your love life until you've completely acknowledged in your own mind how sexy you are and then decided just how sexy you're prepared to be.

You have extraordinary sexual power. It's there—every woman has it. It may be deeply inhibited by your upbringing or your education or one or more unhappy sexual experiences in your past, but it's there. If you can *believe* that it's there, if you can start to feel it, you can gradually develop it to its fullest.

In Tantra, the ancient Indian cult of ecstasy, the sexual power of women was well understood and respected. Women were regarded as "power-holders," even if they were temple dancers or prostitutes, and to have ritual intercourse with a female "power-holder" was regarded by many saints, poets, and sages as a way of reaching a state of ecstatic enlightenment.

Tantriks rejected the idea of seeing yourself as "good and respectable," because that would interfere with your ability to arouse the extraordinary sexual energies that lie within you. In modern terms, that means liberating yourself from any ideas that you may have that certain sexual acts are "dirty" or "immoral," and allowing yourself to relish sex to the utmost.

Unlike Western orthodoxies, Tantra encourages sexual pleasure *for its own sake,* holding that all the body's stored-up responses, emotional, intellectual, and sensual, are fuel for the Tantrik flame. Tantra, of course, goes much further than simply sex. Through meditation, mantra-chanting, and devotional activity, as well as sexual yoga, Tantriks hope to open their whole body to the root energy of the universe.

You don't have to go so far as to study Tantra, although many Tantrik techniques are extremely inspiring and good for your physical and mental health. But you can learn to develop a guilt-free, unembarrassed enjoyment of sex, and your enjoyment will light up your relationships and bring you more pleasure than you thought possible.

Here's Eleanor, 27, a part-time hair stylist from St. Louis, Missouri: "I was married when I was only seventeen. Bob is eleven years older than me. I guess I was looking for a father figure more than anything else, and a way of leaving home. My home life was pretty miserable back then. I was always arguing with my mom and dad and I felt they didn't understand me at all. Bob is always kind to me and gives me whatever I want, but he's very tied up in his work and whenever he comes home in the evening it's always very late and he's usually too tired for sex. He wakes me up on Saturday mornings and makes love to me but it's always straightforward fucking, if you'll excuse me for saying so. A kind of routine. Bob fucks me and then always goes back to sleep for an hour. I lie there and masturbate and give myself two or three orgasms. I feel real guilty about it because my mom always told me that playing with yourself was a sin and that I would go to hell if I masturbated. I don't believe that anymore but the thought still nags in the back of my mind. I guess what's even worse is the feeling that I'm being unfaithful to Bob, because when I masturbate I never fantasize about having sex with *him*; it's always these young muscular studs. I know I'm not *really* being unfaithful, but you know what they say about committing adultery in your mind.

"My favorite fantasy is to go to a college track meet, where all the contestants are completely naked except for sparkling white socks and clean white sneakers. They're all tall and suntanned and blond. Even their pubic hair is blond. And they all have beautiful big cocks and enormous balls, and while they're running their cocks are jiggling around and their balls are bouncing. Whey they've finished a race they come over to the bleachers where I'm waiting with a towel. Their bodies are all covered in sweat and I rub them down, making sure I push the towel right between the hard, tight cheeks of their ass. Most of their cocks are half-hard already, but I take hold of them while I'm toweling them and I rub them until they're totally stiff. I take them right to the brink of a climax. I massage their balls and I pull on their cocks until they're all wet and juicy at the end. Then I stop, because their coach won't allow them to climax before they've competed. It's supposed to sap their strength or something.

"But when the meet's all finished, I go to the changing rooms and meet the guys there. There's maybe a dozen of them, maybe more. They take hold of me and strip me naked and carry me into the showers. Then they take turns fucking me, while the rest of them stand around and masturbate each other. There's jism flying all over . . . most of it over me.

"I imagine that I'm lying on my back and that one

guy's on top of me with his cock right up inside me, while another guy is standing astride me, so that the guy who's fucking me can suck his cock. I look up and I can see his big, tightly wrinkled balls and his huge red cock disappearing into the other guy's mouth and almost choking him. Then he climaxes, and the guy who's fucking me gulps down his jism, and at the same time *he* comes too. And of course that's when *I* usually come, when I'm masturbating.

"If you asked me what my sexual character was like, I'd say that I was a very sexy person. I like sex and I need sex. But if you asked me what my sex life was like, I'd have to say that it's very unsatisfactory. I'd say that it's frustrating. I love Bob, don't get me wrong. But sometimes I wonder how much longer I can go on like this."

Eleanor's problem is shared by many women of widely different ages and sexual situations. She has a strong sex drive and inside her mind she is capable of extremely erotic thoughts. But thinking sexy is more than creating pornographic fantasies for your own stimulation. In spite of the explicit nature of the mental scenarios that Eleanor conjures up in order to arouse herself, she is still very inhibited and guilty about sex, which prevents her from exploiting her sexuality to improve her relationship with her husband.

Many women go on for years fantasizing about what they would like their partners to do to them in (and out of) bed, but because they believe that their thoughts are shameful or perverted, and that their partners would be disgusted if they knew what they were thinking about, their fantasies remain secret. Which is a minor tragedy, because fantasies can only enrich your love life, even if you only talk about them rather than acting them out.

Like Eleanor, many women also feel that if they have fantasies about other men, they are being "unfaithful." I have to say that I have interviewed a number of men who feel the same way, and admit to becoming jealous and annoyed if their partners admit to having sexual thoughts about an athlete or a politician or a famous movie star—or even, as in Eleanor's case, a dozen anonymous young athletes.

It's worth commenting on the male homosexual element in Eleanor's fantasy. A considerable number of women have told me that they are curious about men having sex with men, and some of them have admitted that they would be aroused to see two men "doing it." I believe this is just one result of our increasing tolerance of homosexuality and our willingness to discuss it openly. I have also noticed a heightened female interest in the idea of women having sex with other women, especially at times of crisis in their relationships with men, and at times when they are badly in need of emotional sisterhood as well as sexual self-esteem. But these are subjects we will discuss later.

For the moment, we have to look at a way in which you can liberate your sexual thoughts so that they are no longer repressed, like Eleanor's. What we have to do, in fact, is bring your sexuality out of the closet. You're already thinking sexy in private. Now you're going to learn how to think sexy in public, in the open, where everybody can feel and respond to your sexual radiance.

You're going to learn how to *use* your sexual thoughts to attract the men you want or to arouse the partner you may have already.

Thinking sexy starts with believing in your own sexual attractiveness. But here's Janet, from Baltimore, Maryland, a 25-year-old store assistant: "You keep telling me that I'm sexually attractive to men but I don't think that I am. I'm always on a diet but I still weigh too much, and when I get on the scales I get depressed and I eat more and put on more weight and so I get depressed and I eat more and put on more weight.

"Because I'm overweight I can't wear sexy clothes and I can't behave in a sexy way because I'd just look stupid, right? Most of the time I wear sweatsuits or baggy T-shirts and I don't even think about myself as being sexy.

"Do I *think* about sex very much? Sure I do. I imagine this big guy who's going to pull up beside me one day when I'm walking along the street and say, 'Hey, good-looking, how about a ride?' Then he'd take me for dinner at some swanky restaurant and get me just a little bit drunk, and after that he'd take me back to his apartment where there was a log fire crackling. He'd take off my clothes and say, 'Hey . . .

you're beautiful.' And he'd take off his own clothes, too, and he'd say, 'You're just the woman I've been looking for.' And he'd lay me down on this white fur rug and his cock would be enormous like a big black utility pole, and he'd rub it against my breasts and nipples and tell me what beautiful breasts I had. Then he'd slide his cock right into me, and he'd make love to me all night, until it started to grow light.

"But that's not the way it happens. The way it happens is I imagine this guy, and when I wake up in the morning he was never there, and maybe he never will be."

Here's Astrid, a 33-year-old high school music teacher from Detroit, Michigan: "I had a very intense relationship with a guy when I was in college. Everybody thought we were going to get married when we graduated, including me. He was always very quiet and shy but I loved him for that. The trouble was, he grew up. When we reached our senior year he suddenly found his confidence. He discovered that other girls found him attractive, too, and he really played on it. I guess I can't blame him, but it made me feel like he'd only been dating me because I was the only girl he felt he could get.

"One day I went to see him and I caught him in bed with another girl. That was the end of our relationship, but worse than that, it was the end of my self-confidence, too. If you were to ask me if I think that I'm a sexually attractive person, then I'd have to say that I don't really think so, not until you get to know me."

Why didn't Astrid think that she was sexually attractive? "It's not so much the way I look. It's the way I feel about myself. Some girls seem to *exude* sex, do you know what I mean? Sometimes I think I'm much better-looking than they are. But they seem to have a vibe that men respond to. An *aura*."

You, too, can have this "aura." But you have to start by taking mental stock of the way you feel about yourself and your relationship(s). You have to identify those problems in your life that are inhibiting the free outward flow of your sexuality. You may have had a sexually repressive upbringing, or suffered the unwanted attentions of older men when you were growing up. You may have been taught that sex for women is an unpleasant duty rather than a pleasure.

You may have heard about sexual variations and found the idea of them repellent. Talked about coldly, some of them certainly may seem to be. But in the height of passion something that sounded repellent when you discussed it with your friends over coffee and cake can be the most exciting and stimulating act in the world.

Sybil, 25, a theater set-designer from Norwalk, Connecticut, was appalled by the idea of oral sex when she first heard about it as a young teenager—"How could you actually put a man's *thing* in your mouth?"—and even more appalled when a friend extolled the delights of swallowing her boyfriend's semen. "I simply couldn't imagine anything more disgusting. In fact it almost put me off men for a while because every time I dated I would look at this guy and think, I hope he doesn't expect me to suck his cock, because I'm not going to.

"And there isn't any doubt at all that this feeling made me very guarded in my relationships with men, especially when I read an article in a magazine that oral sex is a man's number one favorite sex act."

So what changed? "I read in one of your books that a woman should never think that any sex act is compulsory, and that if she doesn't want to give her lover oral sex she doesn't have to. And even if she *does* give him oral sex, she's under no obligation to take his sperm in her mouth."

Sybil had learned a vital first lesson in thinking sexy—that you always have the power to say no. Once they overcome their initial reticence, and once they become good at it, most women find oral sex deeply pleasurable. All the same, a lesser proportion enjoy swallowing their lover's ejaculate. "I love the taste but I don't like the texture." "I don't like raw egg white, either." "I make sure his cock's right down my throat, so I never have to taste it." Those who *do* like it, however, seem almost insatiable. "I wish it came out in gallons." "I always suck him absolutely dry, until his balls hurt." "Whenever we make love the normal way, I ask him to go down on me and lick as much of his come out of my cunt as he can, so that I can have a deep, long spermy kiss and not miss out on the taste of it."

The second thing that changed Sybil's mind about oral sex was falling for Rick, one of the actors who appeared in her theater's summer show. "Rick was good looking, he was easygoing, and he was looking for company. He made no secret of the fact that he had a regular girlfriend in New York, but that didn't change the way I felt about him. We made love after the opening night of our first production, back at his hotel. He made me feel so special. I knew that a lot of his charm was just acting, but who cared?

"The next time we made love he tried to go down on me but I wouldn't let him. I felt that if he did it to me I would be obligated to do it to him in return. I crossed my legs tight and lifted up his chin and he got the message, but I could tell that he wasn't happy about it.

"The next morning I woke up and the sun was coming through the bedroom window and Rick was lying next to me sleeping. He was naked, and I kissed him and then ran my fingers all the way down his chest and between his legs. His cock was lying on his thigh, and even though he was asleep I was surprised to see that he was stiff, and that his foreskin had rolled right back.

"I couldn't resist it. I reached out and touched his cock and it was so hard but the skin was silky-smooth. I stroked it a few times and it grew even bigger. Then I squeezed it hard, hoping that I would wake him up, and a drop of juice came out of it, clear and sparkling, and I couldn't resist putting out my tongue and licking it. I know. I was the girl who used to think that oral sex was disgusting. But Rick's cock had such a beautiful texture, and his juice tasted like sugar and honey and something *forbidden,* you know? You're not supposed to lick the juice that comes out of a man's cock but when you do it's totally delicious and all you want is more. And after all, what harm can it do?

"I licked his cock some more, and then I took it in my mouth, all of it, and I licked it and sucked it and I bit it, too. That was the very first time I'd ever sucked a man's cock and I adored it. Rick woke up and he couldn't believe what was happening. The night before I'd been all coy about oral sex, and here I was sucking down his cock as deep as I could.

"I licked around his balls and his asshole and all I wanted to do was eat him alive. I wasn't doing it because *he* wanted me to do it. I was doing it because I enjoyed it, because it turned me on. He ran his fingers into my hair and said, 'Sweetheart, I'm coming,' and that was great, because at least he gave me the opportunity not to swallow his come if I didn't want to. But by then I did. And he spurted his sperm all over my tongue and all over my teeth and my lips, and it was dripping from my nose and all the way down my chin. And I licked it up and I loved it. I loved the taste of it. I loved the smell of it. My only regret was that I couldn't suck him all over again and have another mouthful.

"I really learned something that morning. I learned that if you don't feel pressured and you don't feel obligated, like you don't feel that you *have* to have oral sex or whatever just because you think that your man wants you to, then sex is fun and exciting and it isn't threatening at all."

If you feel inhibited about sex, it's quite possible that you can trace your inhibitions back to your family background or to your earliest sexual experiences. Today many parents are still too embarrassed to tell their children about sex, and even if they do, a high percentage fail to answer children's questions accurately or comprehensively. Jeanne, 31, from Des Moines, Iowa, said, "When I was very young I knew nothing about sex at all. But I heard some of the kids talking about it in the schoolyard. I went home and asked my mom if it was true that men stuck their things up women's butts. I mean, that's what the kids had been telling me. My mom was furious. She said it was the most revolting thing that a man could do and I must never mention it again. She sent me to my room and I felt as if I'd committed the worst crime since Eve bit into the apple. Of course those kids hadn't really been talking about anal intercourse, not in the way that adults mean it. They were ignorant, that's all, and they thought that's what happened when a man and a woman went to bed together. All my mom had to do was gently ask me what I knew and then explain it all. Instead she made me feel dirty and ashamed, and that incident had an effect on my relationship with men that lasted for years. Even after I was married, I was uptight about sex. About six or seven months after we were married, I was having my period and my husband, Paul, tried to have anal intercourse. He was very gentle, very passionate, very loving. But I had it so ingrained in me that it was a filthy thing to do that I wouldn't let him. In fact we had a pretty bad argument. He never tried again, and I'm not sure that I ever want him to, even though my friends say they all enjoy it. All I can say is, thanks, Mom."

Other women have had clumsy or embarrassing first encounters with sex, which can lead to them being very cautious when it comes to lovemaking, and unwilling to "let themselves go." Rosa, 26, a postal worker from Miami, Florida, said, "The second time I made love to Kent [her high school steady], I was so excited that I wet myself. I was so upset I can't even begin to tell you. He kept saying it was all right, it was an accident, but that only made me feel worse. It took me over a year before I dared to go to bed with another boy, and then I was so anxious that it would happen again that he thought I was frigid. It was only when I found out that a whole lot of women suffer from the same problem that I began to feel more relaxed about it. But even so, there's always that little worry in the back of my mind whenever I have sex."

Rosa was right. A number of women find that they occasionally urinate when they make love, particularly if they have been drinking alcohol (which relaxes the bladder muscles and also acts as a diuretic) and particularly when they reach orgasm. There is no harm in it whatsoever, and it is nothing to be ashamed of. In fact several men have told me that they find it extremely arousing because it is a visible and tangible demonstration of their lover's sexual satisfaction—a sign that "I really made her lose all control."

Charlene, a 32-year-old fashion designer from New York, said that she had overcome the problem by whispering in her lover's ear that she was so turned on that she felt as if she was going to wet herself. She rarely did, but all of her lovers found the idea of it intensely stimulating, and when she did occasionally do it, it came as an eagerly anticipated treat rather than a shock.

Wendi, a 23-year-old store assistant from Escondido, California, said that one of her earliest sexual experiences had been so damaging to her self-esteem that it had affected her feelings about men for years. "I was seventeen and I guess you could say that I was the naughtiest girl in school. I was blonde, I was vivacious. I had all the guys after me. All the same, I guess you could say that I was at least half a virgin. I'd done some heavy petting in cars—you know, guys taking off my bra and rubbing their cocks on my breasts, and putting their fingers up inside me and stuff like that. But I hadn't actually done *it*, if you know what I mean. But then my best friend Katie said that she'd done it with Ken, who was absolutely the cutest guy on the planet. I was real angry because I'd been flirting with Ken the whole summer. So I said I can do better than that, I can do it with the Smith twins, like the two of them, both at the same time. The Smith twins were two seniors who were good at absolutely everything—football, track, swimming, you name it. They were both dating at the time, but I really thought that I could get them if I tried. I don't know why. I guess I was showing off. I guess I didn't think that anything would actually happen. But I caught up with both of them when they were driving away from school one evening and I asked them if they could give me a ride. They took me home and I invited them in for a Coke. My mother was in San Francisco seeing her sister and Dad never came home till late. I showed them around the house and then I took them up to my bedroom. I said, 'This is my virgin bed.' And they said, 'You're kidding . . . you're a virgin?" and I said, 'Sure, but maybe you can help me out,' or something like that. I still didn't really think that it was going to go the whole way. But one of the twins started to kiss me, and he was a great kisser, while the other one started unbuttoning my dress at the back. The first one pulled my dress up over my head, and already the second one was unfastening my bra. I said, 'Hold up, not so fast,' but the first one started kissing me again and fondling my breasts while the second one pulled down my pantyhose and my panties. With the two of them working on me, I was stark naked in less than a minute flat.

"They laid me down on the bed. I was scared, but I was excited, too. I suddenly thought that this was it, and that I was actually going to make love to two men at once. The first one dropped his pants and I could see his red cock bobbing between his shirttails. The second one gave him a green rubber and he put it on. I'll never forget that, emerald green. He didn't even bother to take off his shirt and he still had his pants around his ankles. He climbed on top of me and I felt his cock sliding into my pussy. The second one stood beside the bed and opened up his pants so that his cock stuck out of his fly. He caught hold of my hand and got me to start rubbing him. Then before I knew it the first one said 'Ah!' and took himself out of me. I couldn't believe it. He was finished. Before I could do anything, the second one was rolling a rubber onto his cock. He climbed on top of me, too, while the first one came and stood beside me. He pulled off his rubber and held his cock toward me and said, 'How about a suck?' but I didn't want to, so I rubbed him with my hand instead. He was just beginning to get stiff again when his brother climaxed, and that was that. I guess the whole thing from the time we entered the bedroom was seven or eight minutes, maybe less. They just pulled up their pants, said 'So long, sexy,' and went clattering off down the stairs.

"I lay on the bed for over half an hour. I felt like trash. It was all my fault. I'd behaved like trash and they'd treated me like trash. I promised myself that I would never let that happen, ever again."

The problem was that in never letting that happen again, Wendi became so sexually repressed that it was another two years before she had sex with another man, and in all of her relationships "I was such a sexual control freak that men couldn't take it."

There's a vast difference between taking control of your love life—which is the subject of this book—and being so concerned about yourself and your own sexual demands that your relationships are never allowed to develop with any spontaneity. When your lover takes the initiative, you have to encourage it, within the parameters of what you find arousing and what you find acceptable. Much of the time, you take control by *surrendering* control.

Apart from having early sexual experiences that have affected their sexual self-confidence, many women have been abused or sexually harassed during adolescence, and even the least serious of these approaches can cause sexual inhibitions that last for the rest of a woman's life.

Sharon, 27, a cocktail hostess from Miami, Florida, said, "Big breasts run in my family. My mother had huge breasts, and when I was thirteen mine started to grow, too. By the time I was fifteen I was a thirty-six C. You'll never know the trouble I had with uncles and cousins and family friends. As soon as nobody was looking, these men would squeeze my breasts and say, 'My, you're getting to be a big girl,' as if nobody else had said it or done it before. Sometimes they used to give me bruises, but I thought that I could never tell my mother. I thought she'd accuse me of leading them on. It never occurred to me that she'd suffered the exact same thing, when she was younger.

"Men used to brush past me in restaurants and shops, and stand real close in elevators, just so that my breasts would rub up against them. I was so cynical about men for years. I still am, because they still do it. But fortunately I've found a man who loves me for *all* of me, not just my bosom."

More serious sexual abuse can leave a permanent legacy of guilt and anxiety about sex, and if *you* suffer from such feelings, it's critical for you to deal with them as soon as possible. Discuss them with your therapist, if you have one; or discuss them with your friends. If you still feel unable to talk about what happened face to face with anyone, try questioning yourself in the mirror about it, as if you were a lawyer cross-examining a witness in court. Go over the details. Try not to hide anything or leave anything out, even if it upsets you to think about it. Bring it out into the open, and even if you still wholly or partly blame yourself for what happened, tell yourself that it's time for forgiveness.

Other common reasons for sexual inhibition are the fear of becoming pregnant; hormonal imbalance, particularly during menopause; and also the fear of becoming too emotionally dependent. I have talked to several high-flying career girls who do everything they can to avoid intense sexual relationships "because they weaken you . . . you simply can't help it. Women can only have metaphorical balls. Men have the real ones. No matter how independent and tough-minded you are, when you get yourself involved in an intense sexual relationship with a man you want to be mastered. You want him on top of you."

Of course it's quite possible that your problems are not directly caused by a sexual difficulty. Many women feel sexually inhibited because of problems at their job, or worries about money, or overwhelming family responsibilities, such as looking after children or elderly parents.

The essence of learning to think sexy is to identify your inhibitions and to dismantle them, one by one. Purely sexual anxieties can usually be sorted out comparatively quickly. Problems like career or finance difficulties are a different matter and may take a whole lot longer to deal with. But you can teach yourself to compartmentalize them so that they have much less effect on your general well-being and your sex life in particular.

What you are embarking on now is your own program of *meditative self-analysis*. Like the Tantriks, you are seeking enlightenment, but the enlightenment that you are looking for is not the source of Creation but the source of your own sexuality. It's time to clear away everything that has ever caused you anxiety or embarrassment or distress, whether it's something that happened at school when you had your first period, or a disastrous affair with a married man. Those things still count toward your sexual and emotional maturity, but you will no longer allow them to restrict your sexual self-expression.

You need a place for meditative self-analysis, somewhere quiet and comfortable where you know that you won't be interrupted by visitors or phone calls. You need to concentrate on you, and you alone. You need a long mirror, so that you can see yourself while you meditate, and you need paper and pencil.

Although this is not a religious meditation, scented candles can help to induce a quiet, reflective atmosphere. No music, though. You are going inside your own mind, and music will only be a distraction.

Nakedness is essential. You have come to this place to find your sexual self, and it is important that throughout the meditation you see yourself as sexually open, sexually available, and sexually desirable.

"But I don't like looking at myself in the mirror with no clothes on." That was the protest I had from four members of a sample group of six women. "I'm overweight." "I don't like my breasts." "My thighs are too thick." "I'm not exactly Playmate of the

Month, am I?" "Not to put too fine a point on it, I think my ass is enormous."

Feeling that you don't *look* sexy doesn't exactly help you to *think* sexy. But so often it's an excuse rather than a genuine obstacle, an excuse not to take the trouble to dress sexy and act sexy and *be* sexy. These days I don't seriously believe that women who don't happen to look like living Barbie dolls feel that they are in any way sexually inferior. Every society throughout history has had its idea of an ideal woman, but that has never meant that women of other shapes and sizes and coloring aren't equally desirable. Even if you don't have cascading blonde hair, huge breasts, an hourglass waist, and legs that go on forever, you're still as sexy as any woman who does. Your sexuality is *inside* you, and if you allow it to develop, and shine out of you, it will enhance your natural looks and make you appear even more attractive than you already are. And that's a guarantee.

So just for now, stop making apologies for your breasts or your ankles or whatever it is that you think is less than 100 percent perfect. Find a room where you can meditate, set up your mirror, throw some cushions on the floor, and light your candles. Then undress, slowly and sensually, as if you were taking your clothes off for a man you'd really like to please. When you're naked, close your eyes, and run the palms of your hands all the way down your body, feeling yourself, how soft you are, how curvaceous you are, how much of a woman you are. At the same time, breathe very deeply and slowly to relax yourself—in through your nose and out through your mouth.

Before you open your eyes, think about what you're going to achieve. You're going to find yourself. You're going to work through all the problems of the past. You're going to be the kind of woman that you were always meant to be, before you had any doubts about yourself.

Now open your eyes and look at yourself in the mirror. Smile at yourself. *Blissfully* smile at yourself. This is you, starting out on a journey of self-discovery that will clear away the thorns and the rusty barbed wire from the garden of your sexual experience, and bring you pleasure and satisfaction like you've never had before.

Before you sit down and start your meditative analysis, there is one thing you have to do. The choice is entirely yours. But you should enhance yourself with one erotic decoration—just one is enough—so long as it's something that you've never done before, and so long as it's something that turns you on.

Here are some tried-and-tested examples:

Rouge your nipples: You can use lipstick or blusher, or, if you can find them, custom-made nipple cosmetics, which come in a variety of colors—red, purple, yellow, or even black with silver sparkles in it.

Try a tattoo: Try a washable tattoo on your shoulder or your breast or even a more intimate place, inside your thigh.

Necklaces, bracelets, and anklets: Wear bracelets around your wrists and ankles and loads of necklaces. Or fasten one long necklace around your waist and another between your legs, G-string fashion, pulling it up quite tightly so that it nestles between the lips of your vagina. If you use a pearl or a bead necklace the rolling friction against your clitoris and anus can be very stimulating.

Erotic earrings: Attach earrings to your nipples. Or try (gently) to clip them to your vaginal lips as a decoration.

Oils and unguents: Smother your naked body in a perfumed massage oil so that you are beautifully slippery and shiny.

Bridal outfit: Wear a bridal veil, lacy elbow-length gloves, and white high-heeled shoes and nothing else. Remember the innocence and the erotic excitement of your wedding day . . . or look forward to your wedding day-to-be.

Mysterious stranger: Most mail-order sex catalogs offer stretchy black latex masks which completely cover the head and neck, with openings for the eyes and mouth. Wearing one of these, you will look anonymous, like a stranger, and this may help you to discard your inhibitions and see yourself for the whole sexy person that you are.

Change your hair: Alter your hairstyle as dramatically as you like. Pin it up, let it fall free. Or change its color if you want to. Try a wig to make yourself look different. You're trying to look beyond the face you normally see in the mirror.

Titillating topiary: Trim your pubic hair into a heart, or a star, or any shape that takes your fancy. Shave your vaginal lips bare and leave a little plume on top. You can even dye that, if you want to.

Total depilation: use cream to remove all the hair on your legs and your arms and your vulva. Make yourself as smooth as silk, all over.

It takes so little imagination to make yourself into a consciously sexier person. Anna, 25, a legal assistant from San Francisco, California, said: "I love to wear thongs, and I always wear them pulled up tight. I may look very severe in my black business suit and my turtleneck blouse, but underneath I'm wearing something that reminds me every minute of the day that I'm a woman as well as a lawyer, and that I have a cunt."

Melissa, 28, a sound engineer from Los Angeles, California, said: "Two years ago I had my tongue pierced, and now I have this little silver sleeper in it. If a man starts giving me a hard time all I have to do is stick out my tongue so that he can see it, and it stops him dead in his tracks. You can see him thinking to himself, My God, what kind of frightening woman has her tongue pierced—and then you can see him thinking, about two seconds afterward,

My God, I wonder what it would be like to have my cock licked by a tongue like that?"

Sexual attraction is power, no doubt about it. You just have to learn how to accept that you *have* that power. Melissa would be the first to admit that she wasn't a classical beauty. She was short, small-breasted, with what she described as "hips-and-a-half." But she never had difficulty in finding men friends, and in developing good (and sometimes great) sexual relationships. She had confidence in her attractiveness, and it showed. It *radiated.*

Once you've chosen your own sexual decoration, your earrings or your bracelets or your intimate tattoo, now is the time to sit down in front of the mirror and start your meditative analysis. If you find it uncomfortable to sit in the lotus position (with your legs crossed) then simply sit with your legs to one side, propping yourself up on one arm, or any other position in which you feel relaxed and natural.

In normal meditation, your aim is to stop troubling and stimulating thoughts from entering your mind, and to achieve a state of complete relaxation. But in meditative analysis, your aim is to let your anxieties in, and to examine them, and see them at last for what they are: anxieties.

Breathe deeply and regularly. When you breathe in, allow your abdomen to swell rather than your chest, and count how long it takes before your lungs are full. Then exhale, still counting, so that it takes you the same time to breathe out as it did to breathe in. Keep up the same breathing rhythm until it becomes automatic.

Now you can give yourself a body-relaxation check. Are you still grinding your teeth? Is your jaw clenched, your neck rigid, are your elbows stiff? Go around your body mentally, joint by joint, limb by limb, and order each part to relax. Usually, they will.

There's something else that you can do now which certainly isn't a component of normal meditation, and that is to put your right hand between your legs, *loosely,* and start to stroke your clitoris, extremely gently, barely touching it at all. The reason for this is that your meditative analysis should always be associated with sexual pleasure, and an acknowledgment that you are going through this process in order to prepare yourself for really great sex.

The gentle sexual stimulation that you are giving yourself now has always been your birthright, and as you begin to analyze the sexual inhibitions in your life, you should have a constant reminder of the pleasure that you are trying to achieve. Besides, sexual self-stimulation is one of the best ways to rid your mind of unwanted thoughts. Sometimes, at a stressful time of the day, you may find that a few minutes of sexual self-stimulation are enough to help you think your way through your niggling worries.

Beverly, a 31-year-old mother of two small boys, said, "I do it all the time. When I've been working all morning and the boys are having their afternoon nap, I'll pick up a raunchy book and lie on the couch with my hand in my panties and masturbate myself. I stop thinking about Dan [her husband]. I stop thinking about the boys. It washes my mind out like a shower of rain."

As your mind relaxes—as your body relaxes—start to think about the sexual problem that inhibits you the most. You might simply feel that you don't know enough about sex to be a good lover. So many women have told me that they don't like to take the initiative in bed because they're afraid of doing something clumsy or "wrong."

"I was afraid of touching men *there,*" said Eileen, a 23-year-old student. "I'd heard that it was easy to hurt a man if you handled him the wrong way, or that you could end up frustrating him. I didn't want to take either of those chances, so—well, I just didn't touch."

Sue, a 25-year-old nurse, said, "I never knew that there were ways in which you could slow a man down. It takes me a very long time to get aroused, but since most guys I dated were in and out like the Road Runner, I always used to end up frustrated. In the end I was almost put off sex altogether, without really knowing why. I began to think that I was undersexed."

Through meditative analysis, Sue gradually began to understand why she was so inhibited about sex; and through that understanding she learned that she was far from undersexed, and that her frustration was an easily solved problem. She could adopt techniques that could hasten her arousal and delay her lovers' climaxes until she felt ready to let them ejaculate.

The result? "I'm so confident now when it comes to lovemaking. And much more passionate, too. And I think it shows."

If your inhibitions were caused by an unpleasant sexual incident, either something that happened very recently or a suppressed memory from your adolescence, in meditative analysis you will have to search for it, not suppress it. You will have to shine a spotlight on it and see it for what it was. Embarrassing, maybe. Distressing, yes. But more than anything else, it's over, it's past, and it's time for you to see it in perspective.

Jane, a 23-year-old dietician, said, "We went to a neighborhood cookout. I guess I was only sixteen, or not much older than that. I went inside the house to the bathroom and one of my father's friends was just coming out. He was drunk, I suppose, but that didn't make it any more excusable. He pulled me into the bathroom with him and tried to kiss me. Then he took out his cock and tried to get me to suck it. He kept saying, 'You won't want a weenie after this, sweetheart!' He grabbed my hair and forced my face down. I'll never forget what his cock looked like, what it smelled like. I was terrified. He said that he would tell my father that I had led him on. In the end I had to kiss his cock so that he would let me go. But I have never been able to think about oral sex with any man again, not even my husband."

Meditate. Analyze. Breathe and relax. Look at your trauma up close. Take charge of it. It was all over a long time ago, and just because one drunken middle-aged man took advantage of you when you were an innocent young girl, that doesn't mean that your sex life should be inhibited forever, or that you should never be able to enjoy one of the most pleasurable of all sexual acts. Release yourself completely from any guilt, and realize that the blame rests entirely with your father's so-called "friend." Real lovers and caring husbands don't look at oral sex as a way of showing how dominant they are. They enjoy it because it arouses them and because they hope that it arouses you, too.

Sometimes your inhibition may come from a change in yourself, or in your circumstances.

Michelle, a 28-year-old sales assistant, said, "Ray and I were married five years ago. We went to Niagara Falls for our honeymoon. We came home after that and everything seemed fine. Our sex life wasn't very adventurous, I guess, but it was regular and it was good. Then we had Patti and everything seemed to change. Ray didn't seem to be interested in making love any more and even when he did, it was all over too quick. Now we haven't had sex in three and a half months and I don't believe that he loves me anymore."

Meditate. Analyze. Breathe and relax. Look at your

problem from *his* side as well as yours, and don't be afraid to face up to the truth. When you became a mother, did your perception of yourself go through some radical changes? Did you begin to see yourself predominantly as a mother, rather than a lover? Was your sexual passion buried under a pile of Pampers? Whatever they say, all husbands get jealous to some degree of the attention that new mothers shower on their babies, and it's possible that Ray feels this way. Why not come right out and ask him? And even if he won't admit it, make a special effort to give him some good dirty-minded loving after baby's been put to bed. Of course you get tired. Of course you get preoccupied. Of course Ray should be more understanding. But have you ever thought that he thinks the same as you do—that you don't really love him anymore? Look at yourself in the mirror. You're sexy. But don't forget to show your husband just how sexy you are.

"I always thought that my marriage was going to last forever. We were lovers, we were good friends. Then one day James came home from the office and said that he was in love with his secretary and that he was going to leave me the next day. Just like that, after sixteen years. We had a terrible fight, and I said, 'How could your secretary be better than me?' And all he said was, 'It's the things she does in bed.' "

Jonie, a 26-year-old secretary said, "I think I would have preferred it if he'd hit me. He made me feel as if all those years of lovemaking had been dull and boring and unimaginative. And do you know something? When I sat down and meditated about them, when I analyzed what our sex life had really been like, he was right. Not completely right. There had been some moments, like the time we made love in the back of a limousine on the way to the company's annual dinner. I sat in his lap with my evening dress pulled up to my waist, in black lace-topped stockings and no panties.

"But most of the time I guess I allowed him to take the initiative, while I just lay back and enjoyed it. And because I enjoyed it so much I never realized that I was being so passive. After I'd meditated, and analyzed myself, I knew that if I wanted a really great sexual relationship, I had to *work* at it. Sex is a hands-on thing."

Face up to your sexual hangups, one by one, and see them for what they are—problems from the past which you shouldn't allow to inhibit your future. It's time for you to let them go. History won't repeat itself once you've learned to take control of your physical relationships. A really great sex life is all about moving forward—learning to be more sexually focused, acquiring new skills, and using those skills to explore new sensations.

As you meditate and analyze, make a brief note on your pad of each of the situations that you feel you've been able to deal with, and put behind you. Just a brief reminder is enough, such as *"Martin tell-*

ing me I didn't know how to give head or *Mr. W trying to fondle me after class.*

Make some running notes, too, of those aspects of sex about which you'd like to know more—how to make a man's erection last longer, for instance, or how to make sure you have multiple orgasms, or simply how your body works.

Finally, make a list of those sexual problems that you still find too difficult or too embarrassing or too painful to confront. Problems like these will take longer to deal with, but by facing up to the fact that they *are* a problem and putting them down on your agenda, you are taking a positive first step to releasing the full power of your whole sexuality.

And once you've released it, you'll be amazed at what kind of a love life you can have.

Secret 2: Let Yourself Be Sexy

Meditative analysis of your sexual feelings is not only good for dealing with your inhibitions. It's also good for widening your sexual knowledge and empowering you to enjoy all kinds of erotic acts that you may not have known about or that you may have been reluctant to try.

What you should do now is relax your mind while gently stimulating your body. Think about all of the sexual pleasure that you're going to be able to have once you allow your full sexual personality to blossom. You will no longer be shy. You will no longer be anxious. You will never be ashamed of your body or your lovemaking abilities ever again. You will be open, passionate, and willing to try anything.

For full meditation, you need a mantra to chant. A

mantra not only helps you to empty your mind of stressful and irrelevant thoughts, it gives you constant self-encouragement and helps you to focus on what you are trying to achieve—in this case, a stunning sexual personality.

The famous mantra of Tantrik Buddhism is *"Om mani padme Hum." "Om"* is the sound of central enlightenment; *"mani padme"* means "jewel in the lotus" or "male penis within female vagina," the state of completeness, energy-infusing wisdom. *"Hum"* is the sound of power, the engine if you like, that brings the mantra to life.

During Tantrik meditation, devotees often run their finger around the rim of a bell or a glass to set up a soft, endless background tone. This is done as an audible expression of truth—that even the densest objects share their vibrations with the rest of the living universe. But in the case of your meditation, you are concentrating on your sexuality, so your rhythmic stroking of your clitoris will not only arouse you physically but help you to concentrate on the purpose of releasing your sexual energy.

You can devise your own mantra, one that will suit your own sexual aspirations. As a basis, you might use the famous mantra devised by the French apothecary Emile Coué, who developed a form of self-hypnosis based on the repetition of certain phrases. *"Every day, in every way, I am getting better and better."* Coué believed that if this phrase was repeated regularly in a relaxed state of mind, it would become lodged in the subconscious mind, and help to alleviate tension, anxiety, and phobias.

My suggestion as a general mantra is *"I love my body and I love making love."* This has the double effect of giving you positive feelings about your own self-image and also of improving your enthusiasm for sex.

I chose twenty quite different women who had written to me with a whole variety of sexual problems and questions, and asked them to try the mantra over a period of six weeks. They were to repeat it at least twenty times morning and night when they were relaxing in bed, and at the same time they were gently and rhythmically to stroke their clitorises. In this way their imaginations would come to associate the phrase with physical arousal.

Out of the twenty, three reported that the mantra had been "soothing and pleasurable" and that it had "definitely relaxed them," but it had no noticeable effect on their love lives. One woman said, "If I get my husband to repeat it, maybe it'll make a difference."

However seven women said that they felt "much more affirmative" about their sexual attractiveness and "much less uptight about being adventurous."

Rita, a 26-year-old design studio assistant from Atlanta, Georgia, said that she had always believed that her lover, Paul, was more sexually attractive than she was. "Paul's very tall and dark and athletic and I always felt that I was real lucky to be living with him and that there was always a chance that some other, much sexier girl would catch his eye. I don't know why I had such a low opinion of myself. I guess it went right back to my schooldays when I used to be overweight and all the other girls used to have boyfriends and I hardly ever did. I know that I've blossomed since then. I only have to look in the mirror to see how much I've changed. But I guess it takes much longer to change what's inside your head.

"I have to tell you that I constantly lived on edge with Paul, thinking that I was going to lose him any day. And that had a bad effect on our relationship. It made me tense. It made me uptight. It made me much too possessive. It also made me a very negative person, because I was always doing what I thought *he* wanted to do, rather than making my own choices. And that extended to our sex life, too. He was a very good lover in the sense that he was very strong and he could go on making love to me for hours, but he wasn't at all imaginative. It was always him on top and me underneath. And he had no sense of my responses, you know? Sometimes I think that he didn't know whether I had reached my orgasm or not. But I didn't dare to tell him because I thought that would make him angry.

"I did the meditative analysis, like you suggested, and I saw what it was that was wrong with me. I saw how far back my lack of confidence went, right back to my childhood, and I faced up to it, and I said to myself, 'From now on, I'm going to be confident, because I have every logical reason to be confident.' Then I tried the mantra every morning and evening, and I began to see myself in a totally new way. I began to believe that I was just as sexually attractive as Paul. In fact, if I could do the things in bed that I really wanted to do—the things that I used to fantasize about inside my head—then I could be even sexier than him, and make our love life more exciting, too.

"I'd always wanted to try oral sex. I mean proper oral sex. I'd kissed Paul's cock a few times, but I'd never gone the whole way. I guess I used to be afraid that I'd do it wrong and Paul wouldn't like it, but after I'd been through that meditation I said to myself, 'I'm just going to let myself go . . . I'm going to do what I want to do.' Another thing I'd always wanted to do was sit on top of him when we made love. I mean, you see it in the movies all the time, the woman sitting on top of the man, but with us it had never happened.

"When I felt ready, I made sure that I got home an hour before Paul. You said that we should decorate ourselves in at least one sexy way, to acknowledge our new sexy self-image. During the meditation I clipped two diamond earrings onto my nipples, but of course I couldn't wear diamond earrings under my dress. So I shaved myself between my legs, completely, and as a finishing touch I stuck a tattoo of a bluebird just above my pussy.

"I put on this short, black, silk evening-dress. And I mean it's *very* short. And black strappy high-heeled shoes. But no panties. That was another thing I'd always wanted to try, but I'd never had the nerve, because I was worried that Paul would think that I was trying to make a point—you know, like he wasn't making love to me enough, so I had to come on to him.

"Before Paul arrived home I sat down and closed my eyes and repeated the mantra again, and stroked my pussy to give me that confidence that I didn't just look sexy, I *felt* sexy, too. By the time I heard Paul's key in the door, I felt like I was almost floating, you know? And my pussy was so wet and slippery that I could have taken Paul inside me right there and then.

"Paul could sense that something was different. He came into the living room and said, 'What's going on? What are you dressed up like that for?' I said, 'To welcome you home, that's all.' I kissed him and when I kissed him I slid my hands all the way down and ended up feeling his cock through his shorts. I'd never done anything like that, ever—not the moment he'd walked in the door, anyhow. I gave him two or three gentle squeezes and his cock started to stiffen almost at once.

"I always used to shy away from making the first move, in case Paul got upset. But far from being upset, he wanted more, and he wanted it right there and then. He followed me into the kitchen and when

I went to the icebox to take out a bottle of sparkling wine, he couldn't keep his hands off me. I opened the bottle and gave him a glass and said, 'Here's to us,' and I kissed him again and I knew I was radiating sex. I was giving out my whole sexual energy like, I don't know, like a nuclear reactor.

"He held me close and slid his hand down my back and cupped my buttocks, and it was then that my slippery little black silk dress rode up and he suddenly realized that I wasn't wearing any panties. He couldn't believe it. He said, 'What are you doing to me, all of a sudden?' but I knew what I was doing to him. His cock was so stiff that it was making his pants stick right up. I think it was then that I knew I had the self-confidence to do whatever I wanted, sexually. It was like a door was open and light came flooding in and all these choirs of angels started singing. I wasn't going to be embarrassed anymore. I wasn't going to be anxious anymore. I felt strong, and I felt whole and I felt so good about myself. This man wouldn't walk away from me, not *this* me, not ever, and if he did he'd be a fool.

"I licked his lips and I pushed my tongue into his mouth. At the same time I tugged down his zipper and pried out his cock. It was hot and hard and very, very big. Maybe it was my imagination but I'd never felt it so big. I took my glass of sparkling wine and I dipped the end of his cock in it. The glass magnified his cock so that it looked even bigger. I took a sip of the wine and said, 'Mmm, tastes better for some cock flavor.' You should have seen his face. I think he must have thought that he was dreaming.

"I knelt down on the kitchen floor and I took the head of his cock into my mouth and gently sucked it. I wriggled the tip of my tongue into the little hole in the end of his cock and he let out a kind of sigh, like he was *sure* that he was dreaming. I unbuckled his belt and tugged his pants down a little ways, and then his boxer shorts, so that I could slip my hand under his balls and fondle them.

"His hands were resting on my shoulders, and as I sucked him and licked him I felt his fingers tighten. I glanced up and his head was tilted back and his eyes were closed. It gave me such a sense of *power*. I've heard girls say that giving a man oral sex is demeaning but I think it's totally the opposite. You have him right where you want him. And it didn't take me long to find out how to do it. I did what *I* wanted to do, and just felt how Paul responded. He didn't like it when I sucked too hard, and he didn't like it when I chewed him, either, even though he enjoyed my running the tips of my teeth up and down his shaft, just a little gentle nipping.

"I put my head down and nuzzled his balls, too, and he liked that. I could feel them tightening up. That's when I gave his cock one brief suck and said, 'Let's finish this some place more comfortable.'

"We went back into the living room. Paul tried to take over, but I pushed him back on the couch and kissed him again and he didn't resist. I pulled his pants right off and his cock was sticking up like a flagstaff. I took my glass of wine and poured it all over his cock and his balls, and then I sucked and licked it all off.

"I was excited and I was aroused, but I was so relaxed. I had never been relaxed like that, ever before. I felt like I could do anything. I looked Paul right in the eyes with this really smoldering look while I ran my tongue all around the head of his cock. I gripped his shaft so tight that the head was bright purple. I licked his shaft like a Popsicle and then I took the skin of his balls between my teeth and stretched it.

"I could tell that he wasn't very far from coming. His face was red and his hands were clenched and he was panting. But that was when I cooled it. I didn't want him to come so soon. I stopped licking him and I sat up. He looked up at me and even though he didn't say anything there was an expression on his face that said, *'What?'* Well, I showed him what. I crossed my arms and lifted my dress over my head and it was then that he saw that I was totally naked, and my totally hairless pussy with a bluebird tattoo.

"He told me afterward that he was awed. He said he never knew that I could have done anything like that. He had always thought that I was so shy about sex. And yet here I was sitting on top of him, opening up my pussy with my fingers, and guiding his cock right inside up inside me. I sat down on it, real slow, so that I could feel every inch of it going up inside me, and his balls being squashed between the cheeks of my ass. He tried to push up and down, but I wouldn't let him. I just rotated my hips around and around so that I could feel that enormous cock as deep as I possibly could. And I squeezed the muscles in my pussy so that he would feel like I was milking him dry.

"I looked down and I never saw a sexier sight in the whole world. That bluebird flying where my pubic hair used to be. My pussy lips, all plump and juicy, and my clitoris peeking out. And Paul's cock, buried right up inside me, as far as it would go.

"I lifted myself up and I reached behind me, right between my legs, so that I could feel his cock sliding into me. It was wet and slippery and his veins were bulging. I lifted myself so far that he was almost out of me. My pussy lips were clinging to the last half-inch of his cock, and I could feel his little hole, and there was juice dripping out of it like honey, believe me, and running down his shaft.

"He said something like, 'I can't stop myself,' and that was when I slid myself down in his lap and a second later he pumped and pumped and I'd never known him to have a climax like that before, it was like his whole soul was pumping out of his cock.

"It didn't stop there, either. As soon as he'd finished I climbed off him and turned myself around, so that my pussy was right in his face and I could give his cock another sucking. I didn't care then if he licked my pussy or not. It was his choice. But I wanted to suck his cock and find out what his sperm tasted like and see if I could make him hard again, so that I could sit on top of him a second time.

"I looked down and I could see my bare pussy only two inches from his face, with its bluebird tattoo. Even while I was watching, a thin string of sperm dripped out of my pussy and right onto his lips. He licked it, and I could see that he was swallowing it. Then he lifted his head and licked my pussy with his tongue, like he was thirsty for more. The next thing I knew he was opening up my pussy with his fingers and sticking his tongue right up inside me, and licking all around my clitoris, and poking the tip of his tongue up my asshole, which he'd never done before. I loved it. It made me shiver.

"I slowly rubbed his soft cock from side to side against my lips as if I was putting on lipstick. Except that this wasn't lipstick, of course, it was sperm. Then I stuck out my tongue so that I could taste it. I'd smelled it, of course; but it tastes different than it smells. It's *dry*, you know, like astringent, almost. But it has this salty bitter taste that you can't decide if you like or not, but you always feel like tasting again. At least I do. I licked Paul's cock all over that evening, until he started to get hard again, and then I let him roll me over onto my back and make love to me the way he always did. He came a second time, although it wasn't so much of a volcano as it had been the first time.

"We lay there for a long time afterward just holding each other. That evening changed our lives completely. Paul had never understood before what a sexy woman I could be, and neither had I. I did it through meditation. Through understanding myself. If you asked me what I got out of meditative analysis, I'd say, 'valuing myself.' Valuing myself as I was in the past, when I was a fat kid being bullied and teased by all of my friends. And valuing myself the way I am now, a very sexual woman, with strong sexual appetites."

What Rita learned was that sometimes you have to be daring. You have to summon up a whole lot of nerve to make your fantasies come true. But once you've done it, you'll reap the rewards in terms of greater sexual satisfaction for yourself, greater sexual arousal for your lover, and a much greater sense of intimacy and shared excitement. You may think that your fantasies are embarrassing or sluttish. But more often than not, your partner will have fantasies that are far more extreme than yours . . . and more often than not, many of *your* fantasies will be *his* fantasies, too. So could you do tonight what Rita did, and tell your husband or your lover that you're not wearing panties? Why don't you skip the usual "How was your day?" conversation and give him a glass of wine and open up his pants?

Remember that an overwhelming majority of men voted oral sex as the one act that they would most like their partners to do to them in bed. And of course it doesn't have to be in bed. You can give your lover oral sex almost any place at all, and an exciting location can make it unforgettable.

Charlene, a 24-year-old secretary, had a "short, but very passionate" affair with her married boss. "I knew that it was never going to last but I don't regret it. I was feeling bad about myself. I'd broken up with my boyfriend about seven months before and I hadn't found anybody else. I felt like I never would. John made it clear to me right from the beginning that he wasn't going to leave his wife and kids. But that didn't matter, as far as I was concerned. I just wanted to know that I was still sexually attractive to *somebody.* I guess, in a way, he felt the same. I knew that he loved his wife but I could also tell that he had been married long enough to need some excitement in his life. He needed somebody to remind him how good looking he was, how virile he was. The first time we made love was when he took me along to a sales convention in Miami. I don't think either of us expected it, or maybe we did. Whatever, he was a very good lover, very gentle, very considerate—the kind of lover that you'd expect a devoted husband to be. In the morning I woke up before he did. It was a beautiful sunny day and I got out of bed and looked down at the ocean. I was naked, and I suddenly realized that there was this good-looking young guy next to the hotel pool looking back up at me. He must have been swimming, although it was so early that there was nobody else around. And do you know what he did? He pulled down his swim shorts and took out his cock and rubbed it a few times to make it hard. It was huge, with blond pubic hair, and the sun was shining on it, so that it looked bright red. The guy rubbed himself a couple of times more. Then he smiled at me, and pulled up his shorts, and dived back into the pool. I guess I should have been shocked. But the way he did it wasn't at all threatening. It was just like he was showing me that he thought I was sexy. And after that I *did* feel sexy. And I thought to myself, sex isn't scary. Do what you want to do. And so I did.

"I climbed back onto the bed and knelt next to John and started to rub *his* cock. He was still asleep, and at first nothing happened. But then I took his cock into my mouth, the whole of it, because it was still soft, and one of his balls, too. I couldn't get the other ball in, my mouth wasn't big enough. I started to suck him, very, very gently, and roll my tongue all around him. For a while he stayed soft, but then I could feel his cock swelling and swelling inside of my mouth, and soon it was so big that I had to let his ball pop out. He was awake now! He reached down and ran his hands through my hair, and he gently stroked my face and my lips, so that he could feel where we joined, lips around cock. He grew bigger and bigger but I kept his cock deep inside my mouth. I could do that because I was trained to be a singer when I was younger and I can keep on breathing through my nose even if I've got a cock halfway down my throat.

"I moved my head up and down, not very much, only about an inch or so, and at the same time I sucked him, not too hard. Saliva was dripping down my chin, so I wet my finger with it and ran my fingernail down between the cheeks of his ass. I love men's asses, they're so tight and muscular. At least John's was. I pulled the cheeks of his ass apart with both hands and ran my fingernail round and around his asshole. Then I slowly pushed my finger up, wriggling it to get it in, until it was so far up his ass I couldn't get it any further. But I kept on wriggling it, and at the same time I kept on sucking his cock.

"You won't believe it, but I had never done this to a guy before, not like this, not so completely. I had kissed guys' cocks before, but I had never wanted a cock so deep inside my mouth that it was practically choking me. Neither had I pushed my finger up a guy's ass before. I pushed in another finger, and I think it must have hurt him. I could feel his ass muscles clenching but he didn't say anything. I pushed both fingers right up and his cock felt as if it was growing even bigger than it was before. He suddenly caught hold of my hair and climaxed, without any warning at all. Two or three squirts went straight down my throat and my whole mouth was flooded with sperm. His cock slipped out of my mouth and sperm poured down my chin onto his balls. I took him back into my mouth. I was really turned on and

I was going to swallow everything whether he liked it or not. But I think he liked it. In fact I *know* he liked it, because he walked around for the rest of the day like a lovestruck kid and he kept saying over and over, 'My wife never did anything like that for me, ever.'

"About a week later, back at the office, he was scheduled to have an important meeting around three o'clock in the afternoon. I went into his office about ten minutes before the meeting was due to start and I hid under his desk. The vice-president in charge of sales came into the office, and then the finance director and two or three other people. Then John came in and sat down and saw me smiling at him underneath his desk. You should have seen his face! I don't think he knew whether to be angry or whether to laugh. But anyhow there was nothing he could do. He couldn't tell me to come out from under there because everybody would guess what was going on, and that was right at the time when he was fighting for promotion.

"He started talking, and while he talked I knelt up and started stroking his cock through his pants. I have to hand it to him, he didn't hesitate once, even though his cock was growing harder and harder, and he must have been finding it really difficult to concentrate. Once he was fully hard, I tugged open his zipper and took his cock out of his shorts. I ran my fingernails down it and licked it and kissed it. I loved it, it tasted so sweet. And to think that I was doing this while he was having this totally serious business conversation.

"I took his cock into my mouth like I did when we were down in Miami—deep, really deep. Of course, I couldn't take his pants down and push my fingers up him, but I'll tell you what I did. I unlaced and removed his right shoe and pulled off his sock. Then I guided his big toe up between my legs so that it was pressed up against the crotch of my panties. He must have felt how wet I was. I went on sucking him, and while I sucked him I pulled my panties to one side, so that he could slip his big toe between the lips of my cunt, and push it up inside me.

"I think it was a good thing that somebody else was talking right then, and that all John had to do was listen. I licked the head of his cock quicker and quicker, and at the same time I dug in my fingernails and rubbed it, like, *furiously* up and down.

"He reached down with one hand below the desk and clung to my hair. Then he suddenly spurted into my mouth, and of course I *had* to swallow it all this time because he was wearing dark blue pants and he couldn't get up from his desk with sperm stains all over them.

"Afterward I rolled his sock back on and tied up his shoe, and I stayed under the desk for the rest of the meeting. But I didn't let him forget about me, not for a moment. I sat cross-legged with my panties still pulled over to one side, and I masturbated very, very slowly and luxuriously, sliding my fingers right inside. I didn't dare to bring myself off completely because I can't stop myself from shouting out loud when I do that.

"That night, after work, he took me directly to a motel and he was so impatient to have me that he couldn't even wait until we'd reached the bed. He lifted my dress, pulled down my panties, and fucked me up against the door.

"Our relationship lasted—what—six or seven weeks. I was very upset when it was over, even though it was me who ended it. I had to, there wasn't any future in it. Besides that, I'd completely gotten over the feeling that I was homely and uninteresting and that men were never going to find me sexy. I knew I had the power. I knew that I could let myself go, and do whatever I liked, and that nothing terrible would come of it. Totally the opposite. So many of my friends don't seem to realize that if they try doing something a little bit more adventurous, you know, they're really going to light their partner's fire."

It worked for Rita and it worked for Charlene, so why don't *you* make love before dinner, before late-night television, before everything? Why not change your everyday routine completely, and make sex your priority? Not just the routine sex that you've been having since you first got together, but the kind of sex that you've always wanted to try, but never managed to muster up the courage?

Meditation will show you the way to open yourself up, physically and mentally, so that you can enjoy all of the diverse pleasures that sex has to offer without feeling hesitant or as if you're doing anything "dirty" or "wrong" or "perverted." If you have a curiosity in trying *any* sexual act, then try it. Provided that you and your lover both take delight in it—and provided that it doesn't cause either of you any physical harm—then go for it. If you don't like it, you have the choice never to try it again. Most of the time you'll find that your man always wanted to try it, too, but was just as inhibited as you were. As I said in the Introduction to this book, men often need guidance and reassurance when it comes to sex. If you're looking for a full and varied sex life, there will be times when you have to take the initiative, like Charlene. And that is something for which your meditation will prepare you.

Incidentally, it always amuses me that many women still think that giving a man oral sex is in some way degrading. A feminist author once told me that she would never do it because she would never kneel in front of a man—regardless of the fact that most acts of fellatio are carried out in bed, with the man lying on his back and the woman on top of him. The truth is that oral sex gives a woman total control over a man's erotic feelings, and the more experienced she becomes, the more accurately she is able to fine-tune his pleasure, making it last longer or speeding it up. She can even decide what kind of a climax he's going to have, from a deep, explosive eruption that shoots semen halfway across the room, to a quiet, slow and utterly overwhelming flood, for which he may not even need an erection.

Giving a man satisfying oral sex is a considerable skill, and like any skill, it can only be acquired with practice. Only practice will tell you whether you're sucking too hard or too soft, whether he likes to have his cock nipped or bitten or not, how hard he likes to have the shaft of his penis gripped during oral sex, and how quickly or slowly he likes to have it rubbed. Not many men can climax during oral sex without some manual stimulation as well, and only practice will tell you how to balance the ministrations of your mouth and your hand in order to give him the maximum pleasure.

But before you can think of doing any of this, you have to put yourself in a 100 percent positive frame of mind about taking your lover's penis into your mouth. It is no use doing it unless you derive as much pleasure from it as he does. If you don't enjoy doing it, you won't learn how to do it skillfully, and you won't understand how you can use it to vary the pace and the intensity of your lover's sexual arousal. In other words, oral sex is one of the most important and versatile ways in which you can take control of your love life.

If you have problems with your lover climaxing too quickly, take his penis out of your vagina half-way through intercourse, slide down the bed, and take it into your mouth. He won't object. In fact he'll probably think it's wonderful, especially if you make a show of doing it very lasciviously, as if you're licking the most delicious ice cream that you've ever tasted. But what *you* know and he doesn't is that by licking him very lightly and doing no more than dabbing him with the tip of your tongue, you are giving him far less direct stimulation than he would have been receiving inside your vagina, and cooling him off a little as a result, postponing his climax, and giving yourself a lot more time to reach a level of arousal that matches his.

Again, meditation will help you to minimize any reservations that you might still be harboring about oral sex. Close your eyes and repeat a mantra that sums up how you want to feel. *"Every day I feel more and more like sucking my partner's penis."* You can substitute your lover's name for "my partner," or, if you don't have a current partner, you can substitute the name of any man whom you find sexually attractive. Yes, even if it's a movie star.

As before, don't try to analyze the words of your mantra or think too closely about what they mean. Simply repeat them over and over at least twenty times, morning and night, and at the same time gently manipulate your clitoris. When you have finished repeating the words, open your mouth wide enough to accommodate a man's erect penis and try to imagine it slowly entering your lips.

You are calm. You are completely calm. Your man is inside your mouth and the power is totally yours. Sit like this, still, for two or three minutes, and then imagine the penis being withdrawn. Close your mouth, open your eyes, and look at yourself in the mirror. Do you now see what a sexually powerful woman you are?

When it comes to oral sex, some women are worried about the question of swallowing their lover's semen. Semen is only a combination of proteins and simple sugars with very little caloric value. (In other words, it won't make you fat and it won't magically make your breasts grow bigger.) On the other hand, some women simply don't like it (the taste, the consistency), and if you don't like it you shouldn't swallow it, because that will only make you feel tense and resentful and unbalance your ability to control your relationship.

If you don't want to swallow, compensate by doing something visually erotic with his semen when he ejaculates, such as letting him shoot it all over your breasts and massaging it into your nipples, or directing it downward so that he fills up your navel or decorates your pubic hair.

There are many other aspects of sex which women find disturbing or even threatening—mostly because they know very little about them, or they have had them thrust upon them by overeager lovers or husbands. Erotic clothing and underwear are classic examples. Countless men go out at Christmas and buy their partners scarlet quarter-cup bras or black split-crotch panties or purple G-strings, and as soon as the holidays are over their partners are back at the store, exchanging them for something more sensible.

A lot of erotic underwear, I agree, has a cheap, burlesque-show look about it. But you should bear in mind that if your partner buys you something sexy to wear, he is doing it not because he thinks you're cheap, and not because he thinks you're not attractive enough. He is buying it in order to show you how much you arouse him, and that he perceives you as the embodiment of his sexual fantasies. Your first reaction as you lift that filmy piece of black lace out of the box may be one of anger or embarrassment or disgust, but you should think about it twice, even more than twice. Don't take it back and exchange it unless it doesn't fit. If you reject it, or tuck it into a drawer and never wear it, you're rejecting one of his most private sexual feelings about you, and he will shut that feeling away in the back of his mind in just the same way that you've shut his gift into your drawer, and there it will stay forever . . . a small yet humiliating memory of the time that you made him feel foolish and dirty-minded.

Why not *wear* that erotic underwear? Why not *be* that sexy woman he wants you to be, just once in a while? Why not allow yourself to be excited by it? In the privacy of your own home, sex doesn't always have to be tasteful. A large part of what makes sex so stimulating is that you're doing something "forbidden" . . . letting go all of your everyday constraints and inhibitions. We must never forget about romance. But just as there's a time for soft bedside lights and lace-trimmed satin nightdresses, there's a time for wild sexual behavior, too.

I devised an informal test for women who felt that they were sexually inhibited and wanted to liberalize their sexual outlook. I took a recent catalog from a Dutch exporter of real erotic videos and asked them to grade their responses to the exporter's descriptions. They were to mark the action in the videos as: 1—totally unacceptable, in that they would never want to see the video or to fantasize about its content; 2—shocking, in that they wouldn't want to see the video but might fantasize about some of the scenes that it showed; 3—vicariously arousing, in that they would like to see the video for its stimulation value but they wouldn't consider copying its content with their partners; or 4—erotically intriguing, in that they would like not only to see the video but try out some or all of the sex acts described.

The results, although not scientific, were extremely interesting. You might like to try the test for yourself. And, when you've finished, try it on your partner, too. You'll find that a comparison of your scores can reveal what we might call his threshold of sexual acceptance—those sexual variations that he finds arousing and those acts that he might actually like to try with you.

This test has another purpose that I will explain once you've taken it. Choose your response to each description as honestly as you can, and try not to be deterred by the strong language in which they are written. The videos are not arranged in any particular order, either of strength or sexual preference.

Mega Tits—lots of big tit goddesses in full "big tit" sex action. Guys addicted to full tit sex going weak at the knees in front of their dream girls. Breast squeezing, nipples erupting with tit juice, tit fuckers, lesbian tit suckers, tit domination. Paradise for all tit lovers.

Ready to Drop—the best pregnant sex exposé available. Eight months gone and horny as hell! Juicing freely from their hot, open pussies, milking mammaries, nipples engorged with huge areolae. Eager pricks poking up cunts and asses and shooting off all over big, overweight, busty breasts and into pretty faces.

Nympho Sluts—horny bitches who just can't be satisfied. Not happy to be gangbanged by two or three boys, these rampant tarts have to be fucked by up to six guys at a time. One of them needs to be taken by a whole football team!

Arti Gupta—this Asian sex show gives you a fantastic clear-cut insight into the Asian world of beautiful Indian girls being taken in all their wet'n'juicy holes by their horny lovers. Every position is possible in this bid to outdo the Kama Sutra.

American Spanking—very varied spanking action but all culminating in fantastic "over-the-knee" sore-ass spanking sessions.

Nurses of the Men's Ward—very clinical, very explicit. Nurses who examine guys with their fingers and tongues. Doctors who find out about their patients' more personal problems and then diagnose special cures. Nocturnal ward rounds, bed baths, enemas, shaving, uniforms, and instruments of sex.

Boys' Review—wonderfully explicit boys' show. For the collector of young beautiful bodies only. See these gorgeous graceful creatures expose themselves for your eyes only. Fantastic close-up shots of rampant cocks, tight asses, muscular chests and thighs. Treat yourself to an eyeful of X-rated beefcake at its delightful best.

Anal Power—three girls onto one guy. Group sex the feminist way! All these chicks are craving for way-out butt sex. Dressed in stockings, garter belts, and high heels they go all out to claim their just reward from this guy after teasing and sucking him up nice and hard, even treating him to some nice anal sex with their slippy fingers probing deeply in his ringpiece, too!

Black Pepper—fuckin' suckin' soul sisters and big black studs indulging in the best of true hardcore action. Enormous spurting pricks. Cum-soaked and piss-soaked. Proud, bouncing titmeat shown off to great effect. Steamy all-nighters and long afternoon sessions.

Best of Cum Shots—one scene after the next. Nothing but close-up face shots portraying very eager and willing cum drinkers, both chicks and guys. Horniest action with well-endowed big sprayers doing their best to drown their partners in fantastic multi-orgasm cum shots all over tits, mouths and lips, asses and cunts. Twos and threes group cum-splash parties.

Lascivious Lesbos—dripping snatch stuff! Ladies, ladies, and more ladies. Finger fuckers, pussy lickers, tit suckers, asshole pokers, dildoes, dongs, and strap-ons, clearly shown in very wild, very wet lesbian sex. Sandwich sex, bondage, oral, and anal delights.

Punish My Wife—guys who love to see their submissive wives abused to extreme by strangers with kinky desires. Caning, bondage, cunt lips being pierced and ringed. Perverse, degrading torture endured by gorgeous girls with a penchant for punishment.

Dogs on Top—kinky world. The dogs are always keen and so are their mistresses. These ladies are the type who like to "exercise" their dogs every day!

School Girls Like It Wet—perverse water sports display. Lovely teenies who enjoy peeing in the bath or the shower, in the park, outdoors, and more! Solo anal and pussy fingering, dildoes and lesbians but most of all a fantastic, powerful water-sports special.

Thai Bon-Bons—she is young and very beautiful with small budding breasts and a tight hairless pussy. She treats her guy to a night of the wildest sex he has ever dreamed of. Two teenaged Thai girls suck on their boyfriends' big dicks before swapping over and sucking and fucking away with their new partners.

I selected these videos because they are the biggest sellers out of a catalog of more than a hundred, and also because they cover almost all of the sexual subject matter in which today's sex video buyers have proved to be interested. Obviously some of them are what German sex video producers call "bizarre and extreme." But just because you or your partner are curious to see a woman entertaining a German shepherd or a heavily pregnant woman having anal intercourse, that doesn't mean for a moment that you are sexually aberrant, or that you are necessarily going to want to try such things for yourselves.

There is nothing perverted about sexual curiosity and there is nothing unhealthy about sexual fantasy. In fact the more you know about the outer limits of sex, the more balanced your views about sex will become. No matter how extreme they are, sexual ideas are not only harmless, they can intensify your arousal during lovemaking and make you much more creative and responsive.

Jean, a 33-year-old homemaker from Detroit, Michigan, said, "When I was in my teens I read a scene in a book once where a woman had sex with six or seven men. It wasn't very explicit, but my imagination filled in all of the details! I used to think about it pretty often, especially when I was in bed at night and Jack was asleep, and the idea of it turned me on so much. But I thought it was wrong of me, you know. I thought I shouldn't be thinking about things like that. I used to masturbate thinking about all those different cocks. I could hold one in each hand, and have another one in my mouth, and try to take two in my cunt, both at the same time. Then when they climaxed they would shoot their cum all over my naked body, and massage me with it, all around my breasts and between my legs until I came, too. But after it was all over, I used to feel so ashamed. I felt almost like I'd committed adultery."

I assured Jean that she was doing nothing of the kind. If she *were* letting Jack down in any way, it was by not involving him in her fantasy and giving him the benefit of her sexual arousal. I suggested she try to stop feeling embarrassed and let herself go. She didn't actually have to tell Jack all the details about her fantasy if she thought it might upset him. (And only she could be the judge of that. Some men have a very strong negative reaction if they discover that their partners are getting off on the idea of having sex with somebody else, or more than one somebody else.) But she could easily involve him inside her own mind, and with her own actions, and that's exactly what she did.

"When Jack and I made love, I simply made believe that he was six men, not one. When I kissed him I pretended he was one guy, but when I ran my hand down his body and took hold of his cock I pretended that I was kissing one guy but fondling another one who was lying next to him. I rubbed him with one hand and then the other, imagining that I was touching two different cocks. Then I went down on him and gave his cock an amazing licking, and this was another guy, too. I was turning myself on so much that Jack didn't know what had hit him.

He liked it, though. And I mean he *really* liked it! I sucked his balls and then I pretended that there was another guy next to me, bending over, and I stuck my tongue between the cheeks of his ass and licked his asshole, which I had never done to Jack before, ever. That was too much for him. He turned over and climbed on top of me, and he fucked me so hard I thought I was going to faint. I never felt his cock so big before. I was just about to have an orgasm when he came first. But I didn't let him stop. I took him out of me and put my hand down between my legs so it was covered in cum, and I massaged it all over my breasts. Then I guided *his* hand down so that he could stroke my clitoris. At first he pressed too hard but I held his wrist and whispered "gently" and after that he did it beautifully. I had such an orgasm. It was like all the lights went out and I couldn't stop shaking."

Jean's case is a classic of letting go—of learning more about sex and using your newly acquired knowledge to enhance your love life. It's interesting to note that Jean's fantasy was essentially submissive: a woman being taken by six men. Yet when she used it in her lovemaking with Jack she took a dominant, controlling role, right until the moment when he was so aroused that he turned her over and penetrated her.

She educated him. She showed him what she wanted, and how much it excited her, and he responded by behaving much more like the kind of man she fantasized about. I have to remind women over and over again that men are not mind-readers. "He pinches my nipples too hard." "He rubs my clitoris like he's sandpapering a piece of furniture." "He's too quick." "He's too slow." "I wish he'd try another position." But he won't know unless you tell him. And the only way to tell him is by forgetting about your shame and your shyness and your inhibitions and finding your inner sexual self—the real, whole, sexually responsive person that you are.

Let's see how you made out with my erotic video quiz. If you scored 20 or fewer, then you have a very inhibited attitude toward sexual variations and it would benefit you to try more meditative analysis and to question why you have so many negative feelings about sex. Are you still troubled by an early sexual experience? Go back to it, examine it, and do your best to deal with it.

If you scored 30 or more then you are quite well balanced when it comes to sex but your love life could definitely be improved by a little more open-mindedness. You are quite cautious in your intimate relationships and you won't let yourself go with a man until you're completely sure of him. You have some reservations about your own sexuality and the way you look and you need to meditate some more in order to discover your full beauty and your full sexual potential.

If you chalked up 40 or more you are a fairly adventurous woman when it comes to sex and you would be willing to try some unusual erotic variations. You are not averse to erotic videos, sex toys, and dressing up in erotic clothing. However you draw the line at certain extreme sexual acts and you don't even want to watch other people doing them, let alone do them yourself. You have strong sexual fantasies but most of the time you prefer to keep them to yourself.

If you scored 50 or more you are very liberal minded about sex and you understand the difference between fantasy and reality. You allow yourself to be aroused by erotic thoughts without feeling ashamed about them, and you are prepared to try almost anything to improve your sexual relationships.

The hidden agenda of this quiz is to give you quite a graphic idea of how far (sexually) you're prepared to go—in thought, and in deed. Lynne, 26, a sales assistant from Tallahassee, Florida, said, "I never believed that I would go to bed with more than one man. But these two guys gave me a ride home from a New Year's party, and I invited them in. And I guess I knew all along what we were going to do. I went into the bedroom and undressed, and came out wearing this real short nightshirt, with my hair all loose. I'd had a few drinks, you know? And I guess I was a little irresponsible. But sometimes you have to stop saying, 'I'm never going to do this,' and 'I'm never going to do that.' Sometimes you have to throw yourself right off the cliff and say, 'This is the only way I'm ever going to get any experience.'

That's what I did that night. And those two boys were so gentle. It was like they were awestruck at what I was letting them do. And I did things that night that I've never done since, although I might, if I find the right man. Or *men,* even! I didn't think about anything else except my own pleasure. There was one time when I had one of them underneath me, with his cock right up my ass, and he was squeezing my breasts. And the other one was on top of me, with his cock up my cunt, and I reached my hand down in between my legs and all I could feel were these four slippery balls, all squashed together, and I've never felt anything so sexy as that. It was like their cocks were fighting each other inside me, and I think I must have orgasmed five or six times. I totally lost count. They left about three in the morning and I slept for the next twelve hours. I was so sore! But I'd done something important, you know? I'd found out just how far I could go. I'd found out that I was much more sexy than I ever knew. And that gave me—what? I don't know. I guess you could call it confidence."

A full discussion on discovering your sexual self could fill another book in its own right, because every woman's sexual urges are so different. Every woman is aroused in a different way, and stimulated by a different fantasy, by a different sexual taste. Why do some women like to tattoo themselves, or pierce their vaginal lips, while others would never dream of it? Why do some women walk out every day with no panties on underneath their skirts, while others would never go without? What makes some women eager for oral sex, while others dislike it intensely?

It's all a question of personal taste, and how inhibited you are. But now that you're learning to let go of *your* inhibitions, let's look at how you can use your newly broadened sexuality to give your man some of the most erotic experiences of his whole life. And *your* life, too.

The best way to end your meditation is by closing your eyes, indulging yourself in your favorite fantasy, and gradually stimulating yourself toward orgasm. Do it slowly, enjoy every minute of it. Then breathe deeply and relax. Now it's time to shower, get dressed, and go out looking for the man with whom you want to have really great sex.

Secret 3: Teasing Time

Timing is the essence of every pleasurable human experience. Great music depends on timing. Great acting depends on timing. Great sex depends on timing, too. To keep your sex life fresh you need constant variations of pace and mood. You need surprises. You may enjoy listening to your album of Elvis love songs over and over, but you have to admit that after so many years the frisson has begun to fade.

It's the same with your sex life. When your lover feels like making love, does he *always* start by turning over in bed and kissing your neck? Or by squeezing your breasts? Or by sliding his hand down between your legs for a few moments of fingering?

Quite early on in their sexual relationships, so

many couples develop a routine for lovemaking and very rarely vary it. In some ways, such routines are reassuring. A predictable caress will immediately be met with a predictable response. There's no risk of misunderstanding or embarrassment. It's surprising how many lovers—even when they're involved in a passionate, intimate relationship—can still be guarded and formal with each other, especially when it comes to revealing their emotional needs and their most extreme erotic fantasies.

"I'd love it if Anne lay back naked on the bed with her legs wide open and just let me *look* at her," said 33-year-old Peter, an insurance executive from Grand Rapids, Michigan. "Her pussy turns me on and I'm curious to explore it, touch it, slide my fingers inside her, you know what I mean, and take my time doing it. But I know she wouldn't do it. She'd think it was—I don't know. I don't think 'perverted' is exactly the word, but she wouldn't enjoy it."

Had he ever asked her, or tried to coax her into doing it? "Are you kidding? She's my wife. What am I going to say to her? 'Open your legs up so that I can take a good long look at your pussy'?

Although their love life was satisfying, and they made love often, there remained a barrier of formality between Peter and Anne which needed to be broken down if they were ever going to achieve full physical and emotional intimacy. Without that complete intimacy, they would be unable to explore the sensory possibilities of their relationship to the very limits.

I asked Anne if she would ever consider allowing Peter to explore her sexually. Her first reaction was that it sounded "so clinical . . . like a doctor's examination." It's true that a minority of men get very strongly aroused by examining their lovers with real surgical equipment, such as speculums to hold their vaginas wide open. But I was able to assure Anne that *all* heterosexual men are interested in looking closely at their lover's genitals, and that he was doing nothing more than showing her how much she aroused him.

I advised her that if she did allow Peter to do what he wanted, she shouldn't simply lie back inertly. If she did that, it *would* feel like a gynecologist's checkup. No—she should take it for what it really was, an act of love and intimacy, and she should respond to his looking and his touching, and join in. She should stroke his hair, touch his shoulders, and she should also hold her vagina open with her fingers so that he could take a look right inside her.

She should also show him how she liked to be touched, so that next time they made love he could stimulate her in the way that excited her the most. Too many men are unsure how to arouse their partners—how quickly to massage them, and how much pressure to apply. Men grip their penises very tightly during masturbation and they tend to have no idea how light a touch a clitoris needs.

If Anne were to show herself openly and demonstrate how she preferred to be touched, Peter's looking session could very naturally develop into a lovemaking session, which would make it part of their foreplay, and take any formality or embarrassment out of it.

Remember that men are different from women in that they can be quickly and strongly aroused by visual images alone, like the photos of the girls in *Playboy* and *Hustler*, for example. They don't need to know the girl's name. They don't need to know whether they like them or not. They look at their breasts and their vulvas and that's it, their penis starts to harden. It's absolutely natural. And you should take advantage of it. Your lover loves to look at you just as much as those girls in the magazines, only more so, because you're living and breathing and you're with him. But it continues to surprise me how many women are still reticent about exposing themselves in front of their partners, or giving them the kind of sexual display that would be guaranteed to turn them on. One of the greatest secrets of really great sex is using your own body to whet your lover's sexual appetite. And, of course, because it's *your* body, and you can decide when and where to expose it. You can be in complete control.

This is where good timing comes in. Here's Gina, a 27-year-old hairdresser from Miami, Florida, who found that her love life with Phil, a 31-year-old tour guide, was becoming routine. "We still loved each other, but I had the feeling that we were too comfortable together, you know? We made love, we laughed, but somehow we didn't have that sparkle anymore. Phil was taking out three tours a day and coming back full of all the fun he'd had, and I knew why he was having fun; it was because of all the girls on the tours who flirted with him. I thought: It isn't going to be long before he's going to want somebody new."

But as I pointed out to Gina, *she* could be that "somebody new." *She* could be even flirtier than the girls who flirted with Phil on his tour bus. And she had the added advantage that—in the privacy of their own shared apartment—she could be much more sexually explicit than they could.

"The first afternoon he came home around about four-thirty as usual, and I had the whole scene set up for him. I'd just taken a shower and washed my hair and wrapped it up in a big pink towel. When he came in I was sitting naked on the toilet with my legs wide apart. I had squirted his shaving foam between my legs and I was carefully shaving off my pussy hair.

"He came and stood in the bathroom doorway and I could tell he was turned on. He couldn't take his eyes off me, and he didn't even put his shoulder bag down. I went on shaving, stretching my pussy lips so that I could catch every hair. I said, 'Hi, honey. It's swimsuit season. I thought I'd take it all off.' He said, 'Sure,' but he still couldn't take his eyes off me, and I could see his dick underneath those tight white tennis shorts he wears . . . it was so big that the purple end of it was peeping out from his left leg.

"I rinsed myself and dried myself and then I put my arms around him and gave him a kiss. I said, 'How do you like it?' and I took hold of his hand and this time I did the guiding. He said, 'I think it's fantastic.' And I kissed him again and said, 'I can see that you do,' and I tickled the end of his dick that was peeping out and it was slick with juice already.

"I opened up his fly and I took his dick right out. It stuck up so hard and it was beating in time to his heartbeat. I held it tight and I rubbed the end of it around and around my bare-shaved pussy, slipping the head of it between my lips so that he could have some of *my* juice, too, and I had plenty of that.

"We didn't even make it to the bedroom. We made love in the hallway, just outside the bathroom door, right down there on the rug. I opened up my legs even wider than I've ever done before, so that he could see my naked pussy. He knelt between my legs and he pushed his cock into my hole, and it went so far up inside me that I was seeing stars. One thing I never realized before was what it *feels* like, making love with a totally bald pussy. You feel things like you've never felt them before. How smooth and slippery his dick-head is. His tickly pubic hair, right up against you. Your own wetness.

"Before he climaxed, he took his dick out a little way. He actually shouted out loud when he came, and his sperm shot all over my pussy. Thick, white, warm drops. All down the sides of my thighs, too. I lay back and I massaged his cum all around my pussy—you know, really making a show of it, pulling my pussy lips wide apart and cramming my fingers up inside me.

"I swear that I'd never done anything like that before in my whole life and even now I can't believe that I managed to pluck up the courage to do it. But it worked. It changed our love life in one afternoon, and I feel like I'm *released*, you know? I can do whatever I want, like, sexually. I always make sure that I keep Phil interested. Not just interested, I always make sure that I give him the hots. He never knows what he's going to come home to. Like two weeks ago I was wearing nothing but this little pink angora cropped sweater and pink high-heeled shoes. And that was *all* I was wearing, and I used some depilatory cream on my pussy just to make sure that it was completely hairless and soft—didn't want stubble! Phil came home late that evening. I had a great meal ready and a bottle of chardonnay and candles alight, and there I was, all ready for him, smooth and soft and smelling like Chanel. He went crazy. He fucked me right there and then, right up against the wall, and he was still wearing his coat. He lifted me right up and I had my legs wrapped around him and I was kissing him like I could eat him. His dick was totally rigid, and it went so far up inside me that it kept touching the neck of my womb and making me jump and shudder like you wouldn't believe. He had the cheeks of my ass clutched in both hands, and both of his index fingers up my asshole, stretching it wide open. It was one of those feelings you hate and you like, both at the same time. I felt like I wanted to go to the bathroom, big time, and at the same time I was having all these little shivery orgasms. In the end he couldn't hold me up any longer and we finished up fucking on the couch. But it was so great. And I did something else I'd never done before. After he'd climaxed, I went down on him and sucked his dick, sucked out the last of his sperm. It tasted so good! And his dick stayed stiff, not totally stiff, but stiff enough so that I could climb on top of him and sit on it. I didn't have another orgasm, but it was a great little extra, you know? Just sitting on top of him with his half-hard dick sliding in and out of me. Every now and then it would slip out and I would have to push it back in again.

"Last Thursday when Phil came home I was wearing sheer black pantyhose and no top, and he couldn't keep his eyes off my breasts all evening. He sees them every day but you'd think he'd never seen them before, ever. I guess it was the situation, you know, you don't expect to sit down for dinner with a bare-breasted woman, even if it's your girlfriend. Apart from that, I do have pretty big breasts, and my nipples seemed to be sticking out all evening. I don't know whether it's my imagination, but it did make my nipples feel more sensitive, being bare-breasted, and having Phil staring at them like that.

And they were always brushing against something, which made them stick up even harder. No, I don't feel that I'm doing all the work in this relationship. When Phil gets horny, he's amazing. He's very fit, he has a very big dick, and he can go on and on for hours, in any position you can think of. But I guess the guide needs to be guided."

Gina's relationship with Phil had been gradually deteriorating because they had allowed it to become a routine. They made love three or four times a week but always in the same way—satisfying their immediate need for a sexual climax but making very little effort, either of them, to take their lovemaking further. As days become weeks and weeks become months, even lovers tend to take the path of least resistance, and after several years, Phil and Gina were really quite remote from each other, sexually speaking. Neither of them had any burning curiosity about their partner's sexual personalities; or any enthusiasm to find out what the other really wanted out of their love life, and if they were getting it or not. They had passed the first passionate months in which nothing mattered but sex and more sex and the delirium of falling in love and even more sex. Now they were making love out of habit, and failing to realize that routine dulls any kind of human response, especially sexual response, and that there is nothing so destructive to the well being of a sexual relationship as boredom.

Of course it wasn't Gina's sole responsibility to

jump-start their sex life. Phil, too, should have been conscious that their relationship has gone flat and done something positive to restore the electricity that used to crackle between them. But Phil's daytime job brought him all the flirtation that any man could want, superficially at least, and so he hadn't suffered from any lack of doubt in his sexual attractiveness, as Gina had. An exact equivalent is those business executives whose sexual egos are boosted by the flirtations of their secretaries, while their wives are left at home to wonder why their sex lives have become so uninspiring.

Fortunately, Gina was sensible enough to see her situation in perspective, and knew that if *she* didn't do something to revitalize her sex life, then Phil certainly wouldn't. What she did took imagination and bravery. She was naturally modest, and it wasn't easy for her to expose herself to Phil so openly, but the way in which she combined self-display and feminine vulnerability was all that was needed to light Phil's fire, and to remind him how hot their sex life had been when they first met. The last time I spoke to her she reported that she was having "the best sex ever, including something I do to Phil with a very big dildo." She wouldn't say what it was, except that he always had to give the next day's guided tours standing up.

Gina took control of her love life. She recognized her own failings and by her actions she made sure that Phil recognized *his* failings, too. Most important, however, she was always sexy and she was always positive. She didn't let herself become resentful or jealous or sarcastic or vengeful. I talked to a wife in Boston, Massachusetts, who put on some provocative (and extremely expensive) black underwear to stimulate her husband, a lawyer who had been suffering from temporary impotence. "I felt like a whore, but I decided to try it. I wore open-crotch panties and I sat on his face, dammit." When he still failed to manage an erection she screamed at him that he was just as useless as ever.

If she had only forgotten her frustration, kissed him and massaged his penis, and made him feel that his lack of stiffness didn't matter, she could have quickly restored his sexual confidence and eventually reaped the rewards. As it was, they were divorced, and he married a legal assistant eight years his junior who didn't seem to have any complaints about his sexual prowess.

You can put the heat back into your sex life, but I'm not going to pretend that it's simply a matter of walking around your apartment with no panties on, although that will probably help. You've seen how meditation can clear away any deep-rooted inhibitions about sex. You've seen how you can think about extreme sexual acts in order to free yourself from any sexual inhibitions. You also have to be forgiving. Your partner is only human, and what we're talking about here is starting fresh. Forget why he annoyed you yesterday morning. Put aside any long-standing annoyances. In effect you have to wipe the slate and start all over. You have to be that sexy, flirtatious woman that he always wanted: that woman who's loving and giving and willing to try everything.

We're talking about erotic timing here in every respect. Turn back the clock to the time you first met him. Remember what it was that you liked about him. Now think to yourself: What did he find attractive about me? You didn't criticize him in those days, did you? You didn't judge. You never said that he couldn't handle money or put down the toilet seat or parallel park. Your relationship was fresh and your sex was pure sex, without any tensions or complications in the back of your mind.

What you need for really great sex is really great love, and really great love comes from opening your mind, opening up your body, and opening up your heart, unreservedly. Whenever you feel frustrated or let down by your partner, close your eyes, relax, and remember why you love him, and what it was about him that first attracted you. In a long-term relationship, a small and forgivable foible can easily develop into an intolerable irritation, and I'll bet that you often criticize your partner's everyday habits without even realizing it. Your beef probably has nothing to do with sex. It may be the way he wipes the kitchen counter, or forgets to put his socks in the laundry basket. But constant criticism erodes confidence, it erodes trust, and worst of all it erodes that sense of fun you had when you first went out together.

I have had so many letters from both men and women, wondering where their sexual relationships went wrong. The answer is almost always a lack of communication that has become hardened by routine, and a lack of courage to break that routine. Darlene, from Warren, Maryland, told me that she had only six orgasms in the eighteen years that she was married to her first husband, despite the fact that she adores sex and likes to have it two or three times a day, if possible. They just didn't communicate, and at that time she didn't have the sexual knowledge to be able to change her relationship for the better.

Now she does, and she wrote me a very special letter to thank me for transforming her sex life. She also sent me a little list of the pleasures that she has found with her new boyfriend, Bob. "One, we are sexually compatible; two, we will try new and exciting things in and out of bed; three, we communicate; four, we like most of the same things; five, we can be silent together with no strain; six, we can give each other the freedom to grow and love; seven, we love and respect each other; eight, we take an interest in each other's jobs and families; nine, we really love each other."

Darlene said that with Bob, she had been willing to try anything, including anal sex and wet sex. The pride and self-confidence that radiates from her letter is typical of all those women who have had the daring to overcome their inhibitions and their embarrassment and show their partners just how sexy they really can be.

None of them feel that they have surrendered their pride, their dignity, or their feminine rights—even when they've performed a striptease for their partners, or an explicit sexual act. In fact, most of them feel that they've reclaimed them, in spades, because they've re-ignited their partner's sexual interest in them, improved their sex lives, and consequently made their relationships more exciting but very much more secure.

Even sexual relationships that appear in good shape can suffer from what could be called "familiarity fatigue." A couple showers, they go to bed, they watch television, they have "cuddles." They may occasionally try some sexual variations in bed, like oral and anal sex or watching XXX-rated videos while they make love. But a routine is a routine, and routines eventually dull any kind of response, especially sexual response, which constantly needs novelty and surprise to enliven it.

"I love Brad so much," said 27-year-old Megan, a bank teller from Orlando, Florida. "But we've been living together for six months now and every time we make love he does it in exactly the same way. He waits till we're in bed together, then he reaches across and starts playing with my hair. As far as I'm concerned, that's the signal that he's going to make love to me. He leans over and kisses me and starts to tweak my nipples. I can't say that I don't like it. He makes my nipples stiff and he turns me on, but the trouble is that I always know what's going to happen next. He's going to run his hand down my sides, and around my thighs, and then at last he's going to touch me between my legs. A soon as he feels that I'm wet, he's going to climb on top of me and push his dick inside me, and fuck me. I love it. It's wonderful. Sometimes he can make me have an orgasm just by fucking me, and for me that was always very difficult. The first two or three times I was left with this feeling that, 'Wow, this is heaven, I've finally found the perfect lover.' But it's the same every time. We never do it anyplace different and we never do it in any *way* different. He reaches across, he plays with my hair, and then we fuck. You know, I love Key lime pie, I really do. But every single night?"

As she said, Megan loved Brad, but she felt as if their sex life had already progressed as far as it was ever going to go. "He's going to be making love to me in exactly the same way when he's ninety years old," Except that she didn't believe that their relationship was going to last anywhere near that long.

When was the last time your lover really surprised you? When was the last time you really surprised *him*? If you want really great sex you have to work at it. You have to be creative, you have to be provocative, and—yes—you even have to be funny at times. A sense of humor never did any sexual relationship any harm. Maybe the most extreme example of this was Jenni, a 24-year-old dancer from Santa Cruz, California, who surprised her (much older) boyfriend, Rex, when he arrived at her apartment one evening by opening the door completely naked, except for big red clown boots "and, yes, a wild red fright wig, and clown makeup, and my pubic hair dyed bright blue." And? "It threw him at first. He didn't know what to say and he obviously didn't know what to think. For a moment I thought he was going to turn around and walk out. But then I put my arms around him and I told him, 'This is me. I'm an artist, I'm an exhibitionist, I'm a clown . . . this is what I am.' Like, I excited him because I was so much younger than he was, and I was skinny, and my breasts were big and bouncy and firm, but I wanted him to see beyond that. I wanted him to see that I was more than a body. I was more than a compliant young girl who didn't know much about anything. I was *me*.

"He wanted to pick me up and carry me to bed. He always used to do that, pick me up and carry me to bed. But I wouldn't let him. Whenever he tried to take hold of me, I dodged away. It wasn't long before he was getting pretty angry. He thought I was teasing him and I guess I was. I was trying to make him understand that I wasn't his mistress. I wasn't his concubine. I knew that I was having an affair with an older man but I was an independent young woman who had her own needs and having the same old sex wasn't one of them. Do you know what his lovemaking reminded me of? That song, 'Fly Me to the Moon.' Romantic, for sure. Sincere, certainly. But not exactly orgasmic.

"Do you know what I did? I stood right in the middle of the living room and I did a handstand. He came up to me and laughed and asked me what I thought I was playing at. I said exactly that—I was *playing*. I was having fun. Then I slowly opened my legs wider and wider, so that he could see my pink cunt lips opening up, right in the middle of my bright blue pubic hair. And I said, 'You can play, too.'

"He got the message pretty quick. He stood behind me and parted the cheeks of my ass and started to lick my asshole. I love having my asshole licked. Hardly any of my boyfriends have every done it, but I could lie there for hours while a guy's tongue goes around and around and every now and then pokes a little way inside. Mmm, shivery! Anyhow, Rex did that for a while and then he dipped his tongue into my cunt, as far as it would go, and waggled it, and that was gorgeous with a capital G. I couldn't hold my handstand any longer, and I had to ask him to hold me so that I wouldn't fall. He did, he held my thighs, but he kept on licking and sucking my cunt, rubbing his whole face right into my juice like he was washing it. There was so much juice that it trickled between the cheeks of my ass and started sliding down my back, between my shoulder-blades.

"Then I said to Rex, 'Look up, and look in the

mirror.' He did, and I said, 'How do you like your new blue moustache?' And it was then that we both collapsed with laughter. We lay on the floor and we laughed until we cried. I'd never seen Rex look so young, so carefree. And afterward, when we were through laughing, he took off his shirt and his pants and he made love to me on the floor, and his cock was so hard that you would have thought he was twenty-three instead of forty-three. He looked so lean and young and beautiful, I just wished I could have been born earlier or he could have been born later!

"He lay beside me so that he could touch my clitoris while we made love, and it didn't take any time at all before I had the deepest orgasm I've ever had in my life. I don't usually shout out loud when I come, but I did then. My hips wouldn't stop bucking up and down and all the time I had this huge hard cock inside me which made me buck up and down even more.

"Our relationship changed so much after that. *He* changed. He began to have a much younger outlook, especially when it came to sex. I think I showed him that you don't have to be deadly serious to have a great time in bed."

You will have to use your own discretion when it comes to deciding the best moment to spring your sexual surprise on the man in your life. You know him better than anybody else and only you can judge whether he'll be too tired and irritable if you try to jump on him as soon as he comes home from work, or whether he's the kind of man who takes a long time to surface in the morning, and can't even think about sex until he's had three large cups of black coffee.

One of the ways in which you can use erotic timing is to tease him all through the day with several little sexy surprises, so that by the time he gets back to you he will be in a highly stimulated frame of mind. Jan, a 38-year-old dressmaker from San Diego, California, told me that she always tries to think of something to arouse her husband, Ted, before he goes off to work in the morning.

"I guess the secret is to do or say something sexy when he doesn't have the time to do anything about it," she said. "Sometimes, when I kiss him goodbye, I whisper something real dirty in his ear, like 'When you come home tonight, I'm going to pull down your pants and I'm going to suck your cock until you come all over my face.' Or 'How would you like to push your cock right up my ass tonight?' Or 'I want you to tie me up and fuck me until I'm sore.' You can't say something like that *every* day, but now and then it works wonders. He always comes home more than ready to take me to bed and make me keep my promise."

Roberta, 27, a homemaker from Tucson, Arizona, likes to give her husband an occasional flash of what he can expect when he gets back from work. "When he's backing out of the driveway, I lift up my skirt and give him a quick look. Sometimes I'm wearing black lace panties. Sometimes I'm wearing a little red satin G-string. Other times I'm not wearing anything at all. I have to do it quick so that the neighbors don't see, but one flash is enough. He always comes home early on days I do that."

Rhoda, 33, a florist from Darien, Connecticut, drives her husband, Tom, to the railroad station every morning. "Sometimes, when he's just about to get out of the car, I turn sideways in my seat and pull up my skirt so that he can see my bare pussy. I take hold of his hand and rub it up and down between my pussy lips. There isn't usually time to do much more than that, but it turns me on and I know it turns Tom on, too. He can ride on the train all the way to work and smell my pussy juice on his fingers."

Some women give their partners little erotic "time-bombs"—aimed at keeping up his sexual interest all through the day. A favorite is to pack a pair of used panties in his lunch. Men are very aroused by sexual aromas, and this is a way to make sure that he is thinking about you sexually all day. Maxine, 21, a hairdresser from Cleveland, Ohio, said that she wears the same white see-through panties every day for at least three days. "I pull them up really tight between the lips of my cunt and I masturbate myself so that they get real wet. By the time I've finished with them they really smell like sex. I give them a quick spray of my favorite perfume, too, so that John is always reminded of me."

Lydia, a 31-year-old part-time model from Chicago, Illinois, said that when her husband, Raymond, goes on business trips she sometimes packs a pair of her panties in his traveling bag. "He loves it if I've wet them. I sit on the toilet and pee through them. Then I take them off and wrap them in a plastic bag. I know he uses them to masturbate, that's the whole point. He brings them back and they're stiff with his sperm. That's when they turn me on, too. I smell them and they smell just like the both of us."

Jean, a 30-year-old homemaker from Charleston, South Carolina, said, "Sometimes, when we're making love, Lloyd likes to push a pair of my slippery satin panties into my anus with his finger—so that when I'm just about to reach my orgasm he can slowly pull them out. It gives me an incredible feeling, that satin sliding out of my ass, and it always makes my orgasm much more intense. When he does that, I keep my panties and put them into one of his pockets so that he can find them the next day. He says he puts them over his face and breathes them in, and they always give him a hard-on."

Another favorite is to secrete a sealed envelope in your partner's pocket or briefcase containing a sexy Polaroid photograph of yourself. Just make sure that you write on the envelope *Caution, only to be opened in private!* You don't want him ripping open the envelope in the office to expose all of your intimate charms to his colleagues.

Joanna, 27, a bank teller from St. Petersburg, Florida, said, "What I like about taking sexy pictures of myself is that I can act out some of my fantasies, and some of *his,* too, but because I take the pictures in private, by myself, it kind of makes it less embarrassing than acting them out right in front of him . . . almost like it's somebody else in the picture instead of me. What was the last picture I gave him? It was his thirtieth birthday so I did something special. I dressed up in a white lacy quarter-cup bra which shows my nipples. Ken loves that, especially under a T-shirt! All I wore apart from that was a white garter belt and white lacy-topped stockings to match, and white high-heeled shoes. I wore pearl earrings and a three-strand pearl necklace and I curled up my hair. I think it's real important to look classy and dressed-up when you take a sexy picture of yourself, you know, you should look your best. I posed myself on the white sheepskin rug we have in the bedroom, on my hands and knees, looking toward the camera with a real sexy pout on my face like Pamela Anderson Lee. I bought this new pink lip gloss, coral pink, and it's gorgeous. Ken says it makes my mouth look even more inviting than my cunt. I've posed for a whole lot of pictures but I think this was the sexiest. I had three pink candles in my asshole, all of them lit. It wasn't easy getting them in, but I used lots of Oil of Olay for a lubricant and in the end I managed to push them right up. Three candles, one for every ten years, and I was reaching down between my legs with my right hand and holding my cunt wide open so that you could see right inside. And I wrote underneath, 'Happy Birthday! Why don't you come home and blow me out—then you can have anything you wish for!' Don't you think that's something?"

Jane, 24, a trainee accountant from Akron, Ohio, hid a series of Polaroids in her partner's coat pockets over a five-day period, Monday through Friday. "The first one showed my face. The second one showed my stomach—and I've just had a navel ring put in, so that's extra sexy. The third one showed my breasts, and I was pinching my nipples and stretching them right out. The fourth one showed my ass, and I'm spreading my cheeks wide apart with both hands so that you can see it winking at you! And of course the last one shows my pussy, with my pubic hair shaved in a heart-shape, and the message 'I love you all over.' He couldn't wait to get home and take a look at that heart!"

The variety of Polaroids that I have been told about has been almost endless—from virginal pictures of young wives naked except for bridal veils and bouquets, given to their husbands as souvenirs of their wedding night, to graphic portrayals of women masturbating with every conceivable object, from cucumbers to vacuum-cleaner hoses. Most of the pictures are simple "glamour" shots, to remind a man what he has left behind at home, and what he can expect to look forward to when his day's work is over. Like Joanna, however, some women find that they can use Polaroids to explain to their partners some sexual fantasy which would be difficult to put into words. One young homemaker from Lake Charles, Louisiana, gave her husband three Polaroid pictures of herself with safety pins piercing her nipples and hot candle wax dropping onto her pubic hair. She was aroused by pain, and this was the only way she felt that she could make him understand. Ruth, 26, a grade school teacher from Boston, Massachusetts, gave her partner a picture that showed her lying on her back in her tiled bathroom, urinating all over herself. "I love wet sex," she told me. "I think it's so much fun, so liberating. But how was I going to tell David how much I wanted to do it?" The Polaroid, however, broke the ice. "That night, when David came home, he could hardly wait. He wanted a repeat performance, live action, for real. So I gave it to him. I lay back on the bathroom floor and opened up my legs and pissed out a fountain for him. And even before I'd finished, he took out his cock and started pissing all over me—all over my breasts, all over my stomach, right into my cunt. I wanted him to piss in my face but he didn't have enough left. We ended up making love on the floor, wet and sticky and wild like animals." Now, she says, wet sex is a regular part of their lovemaking. "When David goes for a piss, I kneel beside the toilet and I hold his cock for him, stroking his balls. I kiss the shaft of his cock while he's pissing . . . and then I curl my tongue around and take little tastes of piss. Sometimes I let him piss right into my mouth. I don't swallow it, not much of it, anyway, but I fill my mouth right up and then I spurt it all out again, all over his cock and his balls, and masturbate him at the same time. I just love the taste of it."

We'll go back to the subject of wet sex later. In the twenty-five years that I have been giving sexual advice, I have received more letters on this one variation than almost any other, apart from oral sex, anal sex, and bondage, so it's worth discussing in more detail. But for the moment, let's go back to erotic timing, and the "time-bomb" surprises that you can give your partner to keep him sexually keyed up throughout the day.

If you're thinking of taking some Polaroids of yourself, don't be frightened—they don't have to show extreme sexual acts or even nudity. Just be yourself . . . the warm, sensual self that you are now allowing yourself to be. If you want to expose yourself intimately, then by all means do so. But many women prefer pictures that are more romantic. Even a picture of yourself with a sultry smile and your blouse invitingly half-unbuttoned will be enough to show the man in your life that you want to please him as soon as he gets home, and that you want him to please *you* in return. The most important thing is to show yourself at your best, whether you're naked or half-naked or fully dressed. Don't forget your hair and your makeup, and try to choose an attractive background for your pictures, the plainer the better. Look at the ways professional glamour photographers pose their models. No TV sets in the background with trailing wires. No clutter. The center of attention in each of your pictures must be you.

Everybody has a different level of sexual tolerance, and only you can judge what your lover's reaction to your Polaroids is going to be. On the whole, though, they're a very good way of expressing your sexual feelings and letting your lover know what you need. Janine, 31, from Portland, Oregon, gave her live-in lover, Jeff, a novelty Polaroid. She took two identical pictures, except that in one of them she was wearing a skirt and in the second one she wasn't. She cut out the skirt and taped it to the second picture, so that it looked at first sight as if she were dressed, but the skirt could be lifted up. "Underneath," according to Janine, "he found a delicious red-haired pussy."

Jeff's reaction? "He quit work two hours early and came home and fucked me in every room."

The most *artistic* Polaroids that I ever came across were taken by Susan, a very curvy 25-year-old nurse from Riverside, California. She had painted an erotic costume on her naked body with a substance called Liquid Latex, which dries to form a thin rubbery skin. She "wore" black rubber pantyhose scooped out into a deep V-shape at the front so that they only just covered her vulva. Her arms were painted with black elbow-length gloves, and her breasts were decorated with the outlines of two hands.

"My boyfriend went crazy for it," she said. "And

of course the great thing about it is that you can make love while you're still wearing your pantyhose. It was amazing to see a bare cock going into a black rubber-covered cunt."

The only limitation to the "costumes" you can create with Liquid Latex is your own imagination. It lasts for about eight hours and can be peeled or washed off. It can also be mixed with gold or silver "Magic Star Dust" which gives it a metallic finish. "The gold looks fantastic on women but not so great on men," say the manufacturers. "They usually end up looking like C-3PO."

The most *extreme* Polaroids that I ever came across were taken by Valerie, a 34-year-old public relations assistant from Baltimore, Maryland, who admitted that she tucked a set of Polaroids into her husband's briefcase showing herself having sex with her German shepherd dog. "Gordon had been promoted, and ever since his promotion he had been working fourteen, fifteen hours a day, and weekends, too. I was sex-starved. That was all there was to it. I was sex-starved and there weren't any eligible men in the neighborhood. All the men I knew were married and *very* faithful and most of them were working just as hard as Gordon was. So I started playing around with Larry, that's the dog. I guess it started out of curiosity at first. We used to roll around together; and then one day I found myself touching him and rubbing him and his cock came out. I masturbated him a few times and he used to lie very still and it was obvious that he liked it. Then one day I took off all my clothes and I guided his cock up into my cunt. I held him real tight and he was so warm and shaggy and his cock shot in and out of me so fast that you wouldn't believe it, and he climaxed so quick. His cock was thin but it was long and it was very hard. One afternoon I sucked it for him and he loved it, I could tell that he loved it. He lay on his back on the rug and you should have seen the way he looked at me. Afterward I took off my panties and opened my legs and got him to lick my cunt. He didn't quite do it for long enough but I almost reached an orgasm. That was when I decided to take the first picture."

Didn't she think that Gordon would find her behavior shocking?

"Well . . . *surprising,* maybe. But I didn't think shocking. We both enjoyed sexy videos and sometimes Gordon used to bring them back from his business trips and we used to watch them together in bed. Some of them showed women having sex with animals—all kinds of animals—dogs, horses, donkeys, pigs. I have to admit that when I first saw them I was shocked myself. But the women were all so beautiful and they were being so affectionate to those animals that after a while it seemed natural, and I started to find it exciting. Gordon did, too. I wasn't too sure what he was going to think about *me* doing it, but I felt that I had to show him how frustrated I was. I took three pictures: one of us fucking; one of me licking Larry's cock; and some of us just cuddling each other."

And Gordon's reaction, when he discovered these pictures? "He called me at home to say that he'd found them in his suit pocket. 'You're wild, baby. I never knew you were so wild.' I could tell that he was really turned on. I said, 'I hope you don't think that I'm being unfaithful.' And he said, 'I don't care if you are. In actual fact, I want to see you doing it.'

"So, well, that night, when Gordon came home, Larry and I put on a little show for him. I lay back on the bed nude except for black stockings and a garter belt. Larry jumped up on me, and I helped him to get into me. Gordon stood beside the bed and I sucked his cock while Larry fucked me. When Larry was finished Gordon climbed on top of me and fucked me, and do you know what Larry did? He snuffled down between our legs because he wanted to lick my cunt, but of course he ended up licking Gordon's balls, too. Gordon couldn't stop himself from climaxing almost at once, and in the end all three of us ended up lying together on the bed, with Larry licking the last juice out of my cunt. We haven't done it again since, but I only have to think about it and it turns me on! Maybe what we did was wrong, but Larry's a happy, healthy dog, and nobody can ever accuse me of not giving him enough love, can they?"

Over the years I have received several anxious letters from women about their dogs. Most of them have been along the lines of "I fell asleep and when I woke up I discovered that my dog must have had his way with me. I'm worried that I might have contracted an infection." Some have even asked if there is a chance that they could have become pregnant. According to Dr. Eric Trimmer, the editor of the *British Journal of Sexual Medicine,* infection from human sexual contact with animals is almost unknown, and impregnation is physiologically impossible. The only danger is from clawing or biting by the excited animal during orgasm. There have been well-recorded instances of what we call bestiality throughout history, particularly the training of small lap dogs to give their mistresses oral stimulation.

In most countries in the developed world, bestiality is against the law. The majority regard it as unnatural, and an affront to the sexual dignity of both human and animal. My feeling is that all sexual acts should only be entered into from mutual choice, and that animals are incapable of making a choice. From the letters I've received, however, I can understand that a woman's sexual needs and her affection for her pet can occasionally lead to intimate acts between them. But I personally consider it advisable that such adventures remain a fantasy. I talked to a young female stablehand from Lincoln County, Kentucky, who admitted that she had been so sexually stimulated by the sight of a thoroughbred stallion's huge erection that she had given it oral sex ("I mean, really sucked it and rubbed it"). Afterward, she had felt such a strong desire to have intercourse with a horse that she used to dream about it regularly. But it wasn't difficult to see why she was attracted to an animal. She was highly sexed but she had always had difficulty in forming sexual relationships with men—a problem that could be traced back to her stepfather, who had sporadically abused her. A horse would not only be dramatically better-endowed than any man she could hope to meet, and tirelessly virile, but it would be obedient, uncomplaining, and (once sex was over) he could be turned out to graze (which most men wouldn't do). Seriously, though, she needed to address her sexual inhibitions through counseling or meditative self-analysis, so that she could understand why she was seeking sexual fulfillment from an animal rather than a man.

Anyhow, let's continue and explore other ways you can use good erotic timing to keep your lover on sexual tenterhooks throughout the day. Some women enclose sexy audio-cassettes in their partner's luggage when he goes away on a business trip, complete with some very intimate sound effects. ("Can you hear my fingers, massaging my pussy . . . ohhhh . . . I'm sliding them right inside . . ."). One of the most arousing audio cassettes I ever heard was from a young Massachusetts newlywed who gave her husband a long and detailed account of everything she wanted to do to him when he came home—all of it described in the dirtiest language. ("I'm going to sit on your face and squash my juicy cunt all over you until your eyelashes stick together, and at the same time I'm going to bite your fucking dick until you scream. Then I'm going to ram a giant vibrator up your ass, as far as it can go, and stir it around. I'm going to take it out and lick the shit off it and then I'm going to turn myself around and kiss you, with my tongue right down your throat . . .")

The important point is that while these fantasies may seem shocking, they're only fantasies, and fantasies never did anybody any harm. You can use fantasies to excite yourself and to excite your partner, and it doesn't matter how wild they are, or how dirty they seem to be, they're only fantasies. Once you've reached your orgasm, and once your partner's ejaculated, your fantasies will simply melt away. It's only when you try to turn your fantasies into reality that you will have to use more judgment and be much more aware of the possible risks and the probable consequences. Licking a vibrator that you have just retrieved from your lover's anus, for instance, is not highly recommended by us experts, for health reasons. The rectum contains some highly virulent bacteria. On the other hand, I have to quote Tuppy Owens, a regular contributor to the sex magazine *Desire Direct*, who says, "Personally, I get really carried away and feel as if I must have his dick in my mouth, cunt, and ass all at once. This greed drives me to chop and change, so that I get the cock as soon as it's fresh out of my ass, straight between the eyes and in front of the nose, on the tongue and down the gullet, and am usually delighted to detect not the slightest trace of chocolate speedway skidmarks, not a whiff nor aftertaste of poo. I'm always impressed when it's like this, clean as a whistle, and reminded that my ass is, indeed, a sexual shrine."

We'll get back to anal sex later. But at the moment let's consider another way in which you can arouse your lover during the day, and have him raring to get back home and give you the satisfaction of really great sex. Call him while he's at work and tell him in no uncertain terms what you'd like to do to him. Try to make it inventive. Don't just say "I want you to fuck me" or "I'm dying to suck your dick." Think of something that will give him a real thrill, something intriguing like "I'm holding something real big right now and I'm going to push it into my cunt while I'm talking to you . . . three guesses what it is." Banana? Cucumber? Vibrator? Or, "I'm not wearing any panties and I'm going to rub the phone between my legs. Can't you hear me squelching?" Make sure you give him a vivid erotic image that will keep his sexual eagerness simmering until he sees you again. Advertising agencies go to a great deal of trouble to associate their products with good feelings. If they're selling pancake mix or cookies they show a warm and attractive home environment. If they're selling exotic perfume they show a sophisticated woman in a high-class setting. You can use the same trick to attract your partner. If you constantly associate yourself in your lover's mind with erotic ideas and intense sexual pleasure, he will be aroused by you whenever he sees you. By your looks, by the way you touch him, by the sound of your voice.

If he doesn't have much time when you call him at work, leave a single simple erotic idea in his mind such as "You know that pearl necklace you gave me? I just wanted to tell you that I've pushed it right up inside my pussy, and I'm pulling it out again, pearl by pearl . . . it's gorgeous. See you later." Or "I've been massaging body lotion into my breasts, and I wished so much that it was you . . . my nipples got so hard and tingly." You get the point? You have to be *visual* in what you say to him, so that he can see your naked body in his mind's eye.

If he has the time (and if he's alone) you can give him your own version of a sex phone-in line. If you've never heard a sex phone-in line, don't worry. All you have to do is create a sexual fantasy and involve him in it. Describe in detail what you would like to be doing to him—kissing him and running your fingernails down his spine—rubbing and licking his penis. Your fantasy doesn't even have to be realistic. Sometimes, in fact, it's more exciting if it isn't. Your sole purpose in calling him is to excite him sexually, and it can be very arousing to say "Let's pretend." Let's pretend we're sex performers, making love in front of an audience. Let's pretend I'm a dominatrix, and you have to crawl on your hands and knees and kiss my boots. Let's pretend I'm Scarlett O'Hara and you're a sweaty Confederate soldier and you break into my boudoir and lift up my petticoats and rape me.

As I've said so many times, sexual fantasy is nothing to be frightened of. You can use it to enhance your love life without having to act it out for real. Talking about it can be quite satisfying enough. For instance, here are some typical advertisements for sex phone-in lines which are obviously fictitious, but which still attract a huge number of frustrated male subscribers.

"This dirty thirsty girl drinks spermy cocktails . . . he thrust his big cock hard into my mouth and shot stream after stream of sticky sperm into my mouth. I loved the taste and thickness of it, so I savored the moment and drank it down."

"I had my cunt pumped by thirty Cossacks . . . as I let myself slide down the full length of his shaft my cunt made a loud sucking noise as the sperm from the last Cossack was squeezed out onto his tight balls."

"She loves the smell of her own panties . . . all that hot cunt juice, go on, lick my panties. Taste my cum and jerk yourself off while you do it!"

"Hardcore warning . . . I went to the office wearing a see-through blouse. My big hard nipples were clear to see. Then I asked the guys from the office to undress me and fuck me in all my openings. They fucked me all day. Then I took my sticky openings back to my husband and he used me for the rest of the night."

I talked to several sex phone line operators and they all agreed that certain subjects attract far more callers than others. Oral sex (fellatio) is far and away the most popular, with literally scores of phone lines offering "I will suck your balls dry" or "masturbate in my mouth while I continue to talk filth" or "I'll wrap my wet panties around your cock and suck you through them." Oral sex is closely followed in popularity by anal sex, then by wet sex, both submissive and dominant. Sex with more than one woman is also high on the list, as is sex with other people watching. An interesting variation was "cruel wife makes husband suck you and swallow." Following group sex there is a whole galaxy of various fetishes, from spanking to rubber to toe-sucking.

"What men like most of all is to hear about sexual acts that they can't bring themselves to suggest to their partners," said one sex phone line operator. "They like hearing a girl talking dirty, because their own partners don't ever do that, and it really turns them on."

Many of the phone lines advertise that "you will hear words like cunt, fuck, and cock to make you cum in under sixty seconds!"

Talking about sex with your partner is very important to the well-being of your relationship, and far too few couples do it. As we shall see later in this book, you can use dirty talk not only to excite and arouse your partner (and yourself), but also to instruct him how to make love to you better. If you're used to having sex in comparative silence, however, it isn't advisable suddenly to start talking like a character out of a Jackie Collins novel.

As writer Grub Smith says, "If you do that, your partner will assume that you've got another lover. Best to prepare him by making it sound like an experiment you can both try together. My friend Simon was pleasantly surprised when his wife suggested—after ten years of marriage—that they get 'a bit more vocal.' It was, he said, like making love for the first time. Surprising, revealing, and sexy."

Talking dirty on the phone is an even better way to introduce more vocalizing into your love life, because you are not speaking face to face and your words don't have to be followed or accompanied by actions. You can talk much more explicitly and much more descriptively, because what you're saying is all happening in your imagination. You can say things like "When you're hard, you're as big as a stallion" which you couldn't do in bed without it sounding absurd, since he has only to look down at his penis to realize that it isn't even as impressive as that of a small pony. Also, when you're talking to your lover on the phone, your conversation is much more of a game than it would be if you were talking to each other in person, especially if you're pretending that you're a Parisian whore or a naked slave girl or a leather-clad dominatrix. As actors discover, it's amazing what you can find the nerve to say when you're "in character."

But once you've said those forbidden words over the telephone, you'll find it much easier to introduce them into your love life. When you meet your lover at the end of the day, you can whisper in his ear, "Did you like it when I said I wanted you to fuck me?" or, "Did it make you hard when I said I wanted to lick your cock?" (or whatever you suggested), and you'll be surprised at how excited he gets. As writer Flic Everett remarked, "Real sex talk, when you're so carried away that you can hardly bear not to say it, is breathlessly exciting, because you're saying forbidden things to one person, things your colleagues would be struck speechless to hear you utter. Suddenly you're a wanton seductress, driving your man to extremes of passion with your silken, but filthy tongue."

Of course, if you're unable to phone your lover, you can always write him a seductive little note or send him an erotic fax or, better still, you can e-mail him with a sexy picture of yourself. The possibilities for arousing him when he's away from you are almost endless.

Now let's see how you can arouse him to even greater peaks of passion when you meet him again.

Secret 4: Dress to Thrill

After the Christmas holidays and Valentine's Day, lingerie stores are regularly inundated with women seeking exchanges or refunds on red garter belts and black basques and purple G-strings (not to mention bras that are optimistically two sizes too large).

On the whole, men and women have startlingly different ideas about erotic clothing. Men are aroused by seeing their women dressed up in whorish, vivid colors, in fabrics and styles that make Gypsy Rose Lee look like a model of decency—peephole bras, quarter-cup bras, G-strings with holes in the middle, open-crotch panties, rubber panties, black lace play-suits, and fishnet stockings.

Women feel sexier in softer fabrics and gentler colors and styles that are well-fitting and comfortable rather than overtly provocative. Lydia, 28, a manicurist from Denver, Colorado, said, "I've always been very well groomed. I was brought up that way, and that's just me. My mother always told me that it was a compliment to your partner to dress well and look good. I think it's a compliment to your partner to be sexually attractive, too—that's part of it. I wear what I always thought was very sexy underwear—lace-trimmed bras and little lace-trimmed panties. I wear thongs, too, especially when I'm wearing pants or jeans. I would never wear anything old or badly fitting or frumpy.

"So you can imagine how I felt when my partner, Ted, had this package in the mail and gave it to me. He said, 'Open it, it's all for you,' and I could see that he was real excited about it, he could hardly wait. So I opened it, and what was inside? All this erotic underwear—a black garter belt and black stockings, a black bustier that left your breasts completely bare, split-crotch panties, and a black lacy kind of cat suit that covered you up all over except for your pussy.

"I couldn't believe my eyes. I felt as if he was telling me that I wasn't sexy enough. I felt dirty, too, as if he thought I was no better than a prostitute. I mean, this was the kind of underwear that prostitutes wear, and girls in porn movies. We had a terrible row. Ted threw everything in the trash and then he walked out, and I didn't see him for three days. We're back together again now but there's still something wrong between us. I tried to talk about the underwear the other day, to try and clear the air. I was all prepared to say that if he liked it, then, heck, I'd wear it, but he didn't want to discuss it, and that was that."

Lydia's response to Ted's gift was not at all atypical of the way many women react when their partners make them a gift of erotic underwear. "What kind of a woman did he think I was?" demanded Katherine, 34, a homemaker from Boise, Idaho. "We'd been married for seven years and I never guessed for one minute that he thought I would want to parade around in open-crotch panties."

Gaynor, 36, an auto rental manager from San Francisco, California, said, "I tried on the quarter-cup bra, just for Rick's sake. It lifted up my breasts but it didn't cover them at all. It made me look enormous. I've always been self-conscious about my breasts being so big and here was my husband expecting me to walk around with them pushed right up so that they looked twice as big as usual, with my nipples showing through my T-shirt, too. He kept on saying my breasts were beautiful and that I ought to be proud of them but I felt very upset. I always used to think that he found me attractive because of who I am, not just because of the size of my breasts. I don't know . . . I felt like a stripper. Degraded."

There is nothing at all degrading about your partner wanting to see you dressed in erotic underwear. Quite the opposite, in fact. He is paying a compliment to your sexuality by showing you that you are just as exciting to look at as a *Playboy* centerfold and that you can more than compete with other women when it comes to turning him on. Remember that men are extremely visual in their sexual responses. They can be aroused by the sight of a pair of bare breasts or a woman's exposed sex, even if they don't have the faintest idea who the breasts or the sex belong to. For instance, there is a popular full-color magazine called *Slick Slots* that features nothing but close-ups of shaved vulvas—no faces shown—and you can't get more impersonal than that. By giving you erotic underwear, your partner is not trying to make you look softer or prettier or more feminine, which is what *you* would be trying to do if you had your choice. He already thinks of you as soft and pretty and feminine, or he wouldn't feel the urge to buy you any underwear at all. He is simply enhancing the visual stimulus that you give him, and bringing his erotic fantasies to life. He's emphasizing and decorating those parts of your body that he finds exciting—your breasts, your buttocks, your vagina, your legs. He's demonstrating that in addition to liking you and loving you, he finds you very, very sexy to look at.

Many men find it very difficult to ask their wives or girlfriends to dress up in sexy clothing, mostly because they fear the embarrassment of refusal, or the old "What kind of woman do you think I am?" response. That's why they tend to spring erotic underwear on their partners as unexpected gifts—and quite often it's the unexpectedness of it as much as the gift itself that causes the woman to react in a negative way, and leads to arguments, misunderstandings, and resentment.

One man I talked to had given his wife a pair of open-crotch panties over twenty years ago. "She has ginger pubic hair and I wanted to see it peeking out of these little white lace panties. But she was disgusted. She wouldn't try them on and she threw them back at me. I was so embarrassed that I still go hot when I think about it today." It was only a small rejection, and it didn't materially affect their marriage or their sex life, but it remains a sore point after all these years, and "it sure discouraged me from any further experiments with sexy underwear, and a few other things besides." He still wonders what his sex life would have been like if he had found a woman who accepted his gift in the spirit in which it was given. As a compliment, an experiment, and as a harmless attempt at sexy fun. After all, as he pointed out himself, "I didn't expect her to wear it *all* the time."

I don't think I have ever met a man who wasn't sexually stimulated by erotic underwear of one variety or another, whether it be satin or leather or rubber or lace. So even if your partner doesn't seem to show any particular interest in it, and even if he hasn't bought you any or asked you to wear any, don't assume that it doesn't turn him on. It does, believe me. And my advice is to go out and buy some for yourself before your next birthday, when, God forbid, he might just pluck up enough courage to go into a Frederick's of Hollywood–type lingerie store or send off for a mail-order catalog of lacy little next-to-nothings. Even if you're not 100 percent enamored of erotic underwear, buying a few items for yourself will at least ensure that you get to choose the fabric and the colors, and you also get to own erotic underwear that fits. ("My husband bought me a basque that was a size too small. It makes me look like an opera singer.")

Other plus points: If you buy your erotic underwear for yourself, not only will you arouse him as much as you would have if *he* had bought it, but he'll also be delighted and gratified that you're the kind of girl who dresses like one of his most vivid sexual fantasies. You'll give yourself an extra aura of erotic mystique that he couldn't even guess at (even if you couldn't guess at it yourself, up until now). But most important of all, you'll have much more control over when and where and how you wear it, because it's not a gift from him, it's yours, and you don't have to keep on wearing it to prove to him that you don't hate it. You can wear it when *you* want to wear it, when *you* feel like turning him on. Really great sex is just like really great cooking: You have to be in full control of the timing, and you have to be in full control of the level of heat.

Karen, 28, an orthodontist's assistant from Boston,

Massachusetts, discovered a stash of men's magazines in her lover's toolbox. "At first I didn't think too much of it. I think I'm pretty liberal when it comes to sex, and I know that men like to look at pictures of naked girls. But then I started feeling upset about it. Why was he looking at these girls in these magazines when he should have been satisfied with *me*? And I suddenly thought, I'll bet he's looking at these magazines and he's masturbating, and that means that I'm not getting all of his sexual attention. I'm not even getting all of his sperm. And that made me mad. I mean, he didn't even *know* these girls, they were just images on paper, and yet they were taking away something that was meant for me.

"While Frank was out, I looked through all of his magazines—you know, trying to understand what it was that he found so exciting about them. The girls were quite pretty, most of them, but you wouldn't have called them outstanding beauties. Most of them had big breasts, but then so have I. They were showing themselves off in a way that *I* didn't usually show myself off, with their legs wide apart and holding their cunt lips open and pretending to masturbate themselves. Or maybe they were masturbating themselves. There was one *Penthouse* magazine with a girl peeing in a basin and another dipping a candy sucker into her cunt, and I had never tried anything like that. Maybe that was what Frank thought he was missing . . . for me to do a few kinky things for him like that. The trouble is that it's so hard to know what to do if your man doesn't tell you, or give you any idea that he thinks you could be acting sexier.

"But when I looked through the pictures again, I began to see what it was that Frank found so sexy. Not many of the girls were completely naked. They wore stockings and garter belts and all kinds of erotic underwear, and almost all of them, believe it or not, wore *shoes*. You take a look at a man's magazine and see how many of the girls wear shoes, even when they're completely nude and showing you everything they've got. There was one girl wearing black fishnet panty hose and they were all ripped and torn around the crotch area so that you could see the pink lips of her cunt bulging out of the holes. And there was another one with a girl pulling her G-string so tight between her legs that you could hardly see it.

"You know what I saw in these pictures? I saw girls dressed up for sex. If you're completely naked, you could be changing or taking a shower, right? There's no obvious message that you want to fuck. Like you get totally respectable paintings of naked women, right? They're lying there with no clothes on but they're not giving out the message 'Fuck me,' are they? But a girl in a garter belt and stockings and a pair of high-heeled shoes, she's saying something. She's dressed up to draw attention to her breasts and her legs and her cunt and she's saying, 'Come and get me.' "

Karen's analysis of erotic underwear was very astute. What was even more astute was her decision to use the photographs in her partner's magazines as a model for improving her love life. She was convinced that she was just as pretty as any of the girls in *Penthouse* or *Playboy* or *Hustler* and that she would look just as enticing in the same kind of underwear that they wore. "I sent for a mail-order catalog and I ordered a basque, two half-cup bras, three different G-strings, a red garter belt, and some red stockings."

Did she feel that it was in any way demeaning for her to dress up like this, in competition with the girls in a man's magazine? "I think I might have been less happy about it if Frank had chosen the underwear and expected me to wear it. But I don't think it's at all demeaning for a woman to put on sexy clothes to excite the man she loves. Why should it be? And as far as being in competition is concerned, yes, I was, and yes, I still am. I don't want any other woman to take Frank's attention away from me, even if she is only printed on paper."

So what was Frank's response? Karen reports, "I wore the garter belt and the stockings for the first time when we went to dinner in a Japanese restaurant with about a dozen of our friends. I wore them with a simple white cotton dress with big red poppies printed on it, so the red stockings looked no more exciting than matching panty hose. In one of Frank's magazines I'd seen a picture of a girl lifting up her dress just high enough to show that she was wearing a garter belt and stockings and no panties, and she's got this look on her face, half innocent and half really seductive.

"When we reached the restaurant, Frank opened the car door for me, and it was then that I lifted my dress up so that he could see my garter belt and my stocking-tops, and my bare cunt, too. He said, 'Hey, you're not wearing any—' but he couldn't finish his sentence because our friends came up to join us and I had to brush down my dress and get out of the car. But all through the meal Frank couldn't take his eyes off me, and he wouldn't let any of the other guys get anywhere near me. He hadn't been so possessive since we first went out together. One of my friends couldn't help noticing. She said, 'It's incredible the way that Frank still has the hots for you, after all this time.' And it was a strange thing, because wearing that underwear made *me* feel sexier, too. In fact I could hardly wait to get Frank back home. My cunt was juicy and of course I could feel it because I wasn't wearing any panties and the restaurant's air-conditioning was turned on full!

"As it turned out, neither of us could wait until we got home. We turned off the main highway down this track that leads through the woods. Frank took hold of me and kissed me like he wanted to eat me. He ran his hands up my thighs and touched the bare skin above my stocking-tops. Then he slid his fingers into the tops of my stockings and said, 'These are sensational. I never knew you wore these.' He squeezed and caressed my bottom, and then I opened my legs a little so that he could touch my cunt. He could feel how juicy I was and he stroked my clitoris and my lips a little and then he slid his middle finger right up inside me.

"I needed him so bad I opened up his zipper and took out his cock. It was incredibly hard and it was almost as juicy as my cunt was. I could smell that wonderful male smell, too. The smell of cock always turned me on. I ducked my head down and sucked it, running my tongue all the way around it. Then I lifted my dress right up and I climbed onto his lap. I held his cock in my hand and positioned it right between the lips of my cunt. I sat down on it, very, very slow, even though I wanted it fast. I guess I was teasing myself as much as him. And there was that wonderful feeling of a huge hard cock sliding up inside me, farther and farther. Frank kissed me again and fondled my breasts through my dress and said, 'You're amazing. You surprise me more and more each day.' I have to say that I amazed myself. Wearing those stockings and that garter belt turned Frank on, but it turned me on just as much. I felt like I was able to arouse him. I felt like I was in charge. I sat in his lap and I went up and down at my own speed, even though he kept trying to fuck me faster. Whenever he went too fast, I just lifted up my hips so that his cock was scarcely inside me at all, just his cock head between my lips, and when he slowed down I sank right down so that he was buried in me.

"He lasted much longer than he usually did. He twisted his hands into my garters and he gripped my hips tight and he rammed himself into me so deep that he made me shout out loud. I guess there were a few startled deer in those woods that night! His cock felt huge, much bigger than usual, but that might just have been me, because my cunt kept going into amazing spasms, like tiny orgasms, one after another, which were heaven, each one of them was heaven, but not quite enough to satisfy me completely. He said, 'You're such a temptress. You're so fucking wonderful. I love fucking you so much.' Then he gritted his teeth and said, "Oh-oh-oh-oh-oh . . ." and I could feel his cock head bulge and all of his warm sperm pumping into me.

"Headlights were coming down the track and I was worried that it might be the police so I climbed off Frank's lap. His cock was red from fucking so hard and it was still half stiff. A drip of sperm slid out of my cunt and ran down my thigh onto my stocking-top. Another drop slid out of Frank's cock. I wiped it off with my hand then I licked my fingers. Delicious! Then I pushed his cock back into his pants and zippered him up before the other driver came any closer. As it turned out, it was an old man looking for his dog. But it turned me on to sit talking to him with no panties on and my stockings wet with sperm. If only he'd known!

"When we got back home we went straight to the bedroom. Frank undressed so fast it was like a magic act. I took off my dress, but I left on my garter belt and my stockings and my shoes. Frank was amazed that I left my shoes on, but it's incredible how sexy it is, making love in a pair of red high heels. Frank couldn't get enough of me. He wanted to climb on top of me and start fucking me right away, but I said no. He couldn't have me again until he'd licked my cunt clean from the last time. Now I had *never* said anything to him like that before. I don't think I would have dared. But he wanted me so much, he was so much under my spell, that I think he would have done anything for me, anything at all, and that gave me the power and the confidence. And it felt so good.

"He opened my thighs and he started to kiss my cunt. He licked all around it and he flicked at my clitoris. I reached down with both hands and stretched my cunt lips wide apart, like the girls in the magazines. I could feel his sperm pouring out of my cunt and sliding down between the cheeks of my ass. Frank hesitated for a moment, and then he licked his sperm off my anus, and gradually started licking a little higher and a little higher until he was licking it right out of my cunt like a cat licking up cream. He looked up at me and he had his own sperm running down his chin and a thin string of it joining the tip of his tongue to my cunt. That was so sexy that I said, 'You can fuck me now,' because I absolutely had to have his cock inside me. And of course when he kissed me I had all that delicious taste of sperm.

"All I can say is that my underwear worked wonders. And my shoes, too. While he was fucking me I dug my heels into him, and then I wound my legs around his waist. He fucked me harder and harder until he was panting too much to speak. The veins in his cock were standing out like ropes and his balls were crunched tight. I took off one of my shoes. I reached down between my legs so that my fingers were slippery with juice and I rubbed it on the heel. Then I spread the cheeks of his ass and slowly pushed the heel into his anus, until it was up as far as it could go, with the rest of the shoe 'standing' on his balls.

"He had such a climax he couldn't stop shaking; and then I did, too, an amazing blackout of an orgasm, and for ages and ages afterward we couldn't even speak. In the end I said, 'So you like my stockings?'

"I don't wear them very often—either the stockings or the other underwear that I bought, which Frank adores, too. But I'd say to any woman who wants to spice up her sex life that erotic underwear sure doesn't do it any harm."

A brief warning—if you are going to insert any object into your lover's anus, it is not advisable to follow Karen's example and use the heel of one of your shoes. There is a risk of infection from anything as dirty as the bottom of a shoe, and there is also a very real danger that an object so rigid and sharp-edged could damage the delicate rectal tissues or even perforate the wall of the rectum, with very serious consequences. These days, you can enjoy giving and receiving anal stimulation with any number of anal probes and so-called "butt plugs," some of which inflate and many of which vibrate, but all of which are made of smooth, pliable materials and specially designed not to get accidentally lost inside the rectum—which can necessitate an embarrassing visit to the ER. With care, and with plenty of KY or other suitable lubricant, you can improvise with carrots or suitably shaped plastic bottles or containers. One 36-year-old woman from Fort Lauderdale, Florida, had "trained" her husband with a succession of larger and larger candles, until he could take an altar candle three inches in diameter into his anus, to a depth of more than seven inches. "When I do that, his climaxes shoot clear across the room."

Where you wear your sexy clothing is almost as important as the clothing itself. Karen gave Frank a quick flash of her garter belt and stockings in the car, which was much more erotic than merely strolling into the bedroom wearing them. So whatever you decide to wear (or whatever you decide *not* to wear), make sure that you pick your moment. If he is unable to make love to you immediately—for instance, if you breathe into his ear in a crowded street, 'I'm wearing tight black rubber panties under my skirt'—you will greatly increase his sexual tension and give him that much longer to work up a lather of sexual anticipation.

You don't necessarily have to dress like a stripper to arouse your man. If you really don't think that you can bring yourself to wear G-strings and basques, or you don't think that you have the figure for them, you can still appear stunningly sexy in your everyday clothes.

Gemma, 27, from Fort Worth, Texas, was self-conscious about her small breasts and even more concerned about them after she had finished breast-feeding her second son. Her husband, Nolan, "wouldn't leave my breasts alone" when they were swollen with milk. But later he seemed to lose interest in them during foreplay and Gemma's love life "wasn't at all what it used to be . . . it's just in and out and that's it."

Gemma could have revived Nolan's sexual interest in several ways. One would have been to buy a bra that gave her more uplift and a more defined cleavage, and unbutton her blouses and her shirts a little lower. Another way would have been to try a quarter-cup bra, which would give her uplift but leave her nipples completely exposed. Then again, with a very small bust, she could have gone without a bra altogether, and made sure that Nolan was aware of it by wearing tight T-shirts or see-through blouses or (again) unbuttoning her shirts. If she'd had the confidence to do it openly, and in company, she could well have been surprised by a sudden improvement in his sexual attentiveness. There is nothing like a little jealousy to refocus a man's attention on his partner.

Gemma had even been thinking about breast enlargement, but I always advise women to be very cautious about looking for a surgical solution to an emotional problem. Breast enlargement is all very well if your sexual relationship is in good shape and it's something that you really want to do for your own self-enhancement. Some women enjoy having enormous breasts and the attention that it brings them. Look at the pantheon of strippers with names like Melissa Mounds and Tracey Topps and Busty Belle. But women who enlarge their breasts simply in order to revive their partner's sexual interest in them are often very disappointed. Relationships go off-track for all kinds of reasons, some of which are not as obvious as a small bust.

Nolan must have been sexually attracted to Gemma when he first met her—attracted enough to eventually marry her and to have a child with her. Obviously he was pleased and aroused by the increase in the size of Gemma's breasts when she became pregnant, but this reaction is more complex than sheer size. Men feel a strong sexual pride in seeing their partner's breasts grow bigger and their stomach swelling. It's a little bit of Tarzan-like chest-thumping—"Look what a man I am. I've had sex with this beautiful woman and made her pregnant." Also, many men find pregnant women extremely erotic. These days, you can buy any number of pornographic magazines and videos featuring pregnant and lactating women, and this is nothing new. Pregnant women have been depicted throughout history in erotic drawings and paintings—such as the memorable "X-Ray" drawing by the German artist Hans Bellmer, showing the interior of a pregnant woman being simultaneously penetrated by two men, vaginally and anally, while a third man forces his penis down her throat.

A pregnant woman has a sexual aura about her that men find both arousing and alarming.

After pregnancy, however, it is not just a woman's body that changes, it is the whole balance of her relationship with her partner. Gemma said that Nolan showed no obvious signs of being jealous of their new baby, but the arrival of a child inevitably reduces the amount of time and attention that a woman can give to the man in her life, and for some men (even though they put a brave face on it) this can be emotionally disorienting and sexually frustrating. "One day I came first. Then the baby came first. She was right on the brink of an orgasm and the baby started crying and that was it. She was out of bed like a jackrabbit."

Toward the end of a pregnancy, most couples tend to have far less sex than usual, and sometimes, on their gynecologist's advice, no sex at all. But if a man is expecting that as soon as the baby is born, he will immediately be able to resume normal relations, he will usually be disappointed. Suddenly he is no longer the sole object of his partner's affections; and his partner is distracted and tired, especially if she is breastfeeding. More than one husband has told me, "My wife's breasts were *mine,* do you know what I mean? I was the only one who could touch them. I was the only one who could touch them and kiss them. All of a sudden here was this baby sucking them for lunch, and she didn't want me to touch them because they were sore. I tried to tell myself to be mature, that this was my child, too. I never said a word to my wife. But secretly I still resented it."

In the first few weeks after delivery, a woman will have far less interest in prolonged, passionate lovemaking sessions, and it is now that many sexual relationships become extremely strained. The man is expecting his sexual dues after weeks of abstinence. The woman is looking for support, comfort, security, yes, and sex, too, but deep, reassuring, affectionate sex, not swinging-from-the-chandelier sex.

It was my feeling that Nolan's lovemaking had become a matter of "whip-it-in-and-whip-it-out" not because of the reduced size of Gemma's breasts but because he felt that she wasn't paying full attention to his sexual needs. He was having sex with her simply to get his rocks off—and as quickly as possible. There may even have been an element of revenge in what he was doing—"you're not paying any attention to me so I'm not going to pay any attention to you"—which is childish, certainly, but it happens in all kinds of relationships and for all kinds of different reasons.

Nolan should have come out and told Gemma how he felt and Gemma, for her part, should have found a way to keep him sexually stimulated and sexually satisfied without necessarily indulging in the athletic intercourse that they had been used to. All that would come back, once the baby was older and everything had settled down, but being a man, and being a very frustrated man, he wasn't to know that. It was up to Gemma to make sure that she aroused him now and gave him some idea of what sexual delights he could expect in the very near future, when the disruption of having a baby had died down.

I suggested that she dress and behave in a way that drew attention to the one part of her body about which she felt the least confident—her breasts. Although her baby was on formula by the time she got in touch with me, she had breastfed for three weeks after the birth, and it seemed very likely that Nolan was still suffering a hangover from the old breast jealousy problem. You can laugh about it, but it's the way that men feel.

"Nolan doesn't work Wednesdays, so I got up early when he was still asleep. Most mornings Ryan [their baby] sleeps till nine o'clock so I didn't have to worry about him. I put on my cut-off denim shorts and that was all. It felt kind of strange walking around the house bare-breasted because I usually wear a baggy T- shirt or something. But I thought it was pretty sexy. I looked at myself in the mirror in the hallway and I squeezed my breasts and pushed them up a bit with my hands and I thought, Gemma, you have beautiful breasts, let's make sure that Nolan takes notice of them.

"I went into the kitchen and made some coffee and some pancakes. It didn't take long to get used to the feeling of being half-naked. I began to enjoy it. It began to feel natural. I took the coffee and the pancakes into the bedroom and sat down on the edge of the bed and shook Nolan awake. I said, 'Hey, breakfast.' He opened his eyes and said, 'Great . . .' and then he opened his eyes even wider and said, 'Heyy . . . what's this?' I said, 'Topless breakfast service. Any complaints?' And he just shrugged and smiled and I don't think he could believe it.

"I poured him some coffee and put it on the nightstand. Then I picked up the syrup bottle, but I didn't pour it over his pancakes. I poured it over my breasts, so that it dripped off my nipples, and then I put down the bottle and smeared the syrup around and around, all over my breasts. I said, 'If you want syrup on your pancakes, this is where you can get it from.'

"He didn't hesitate. And that's when I knew that everything was going to be okay between us. He set his breakfast tray to one side and he leaned forward and he started to lick that syrup off my breasts. His tongue went around and around my nipples until they were sticking up so hard! Then he took my nipples between his teeth and gently stretched them out, and chewed them, and licked them, and sucked the last drop of syrup off them.

"He said, 'This can't stop here.' He kept on kissing my breasts while he unfastened my shorts. He tugged them off me and threw them across the room. He said, 'Kneel on the bed, that's it, hands and knees,' and I did, and we were both laughing because it was so sexy and such fun, you know, we were acting the way we used to act before we had Ryan. This was us, the way we were.

"He opened up the cheeks of my ass and he slowly poured syrup onto my asshole. He pushed his finger inside, right up to the knuckle, and then he took it out again and sucked it, and said, 'You always had the sweetest ass in town.' He turned me over and opened my legs up wide. It was the first time that he'd really taken a look at my cunt in daylight since Ryan was born, and that meant something to me because he was looking at it as something that turned him on, instead of the hole that Ryan had come out of. My cunt was completely hairless. They shaved it when I was in delivery, and I liked it so much that I kept on using a depilatory once or twice a week so that my hair never grew back. Nolan poured syrup all over my cunt lips, and massaged my clitoris with it. He opened up my lips and poured more syrup right into my cunt hole. It slid out all over the sheets, every which way.

"His dick was sticking out of his shorts. I held it tight and I rubbed it, and then I pulled his shorts down around his knees. I took the syrup bottle away from him and I poured syrup all over the head of his cock. I slid underneath him a little ways, and then I massaged his syrupy cock against my nipples. My nipples were so stiff that I could push them into the hole at the end of his cock. I massaged syrup all around his balls, around and around, and then I slid even farther down the bed and took his balls into my mouth and licked them, and licked his asshole, too. I hadn't even done that before and I wanted more. I slid right under him, between his legs, and while he knelt on the bed I pulled apart the cheeks of his ass and gave his asshole a long, slow licking. I never knew before then how much men like having their assholes licked . . . well, Nolan certainly does. I rolled up my tongue and managed to push it a little way inside and all he could say was 'Baby, baby, baby . . .'

"After a while he rolled over onto his back and I knew that he wanted to make love to me, but I remembered what you said about concentrating on my breasts. I knelt between his legs and took that huge sticky cock in my hands and I opened my mouth and I took it so far down my throat that I almost choked. I sucked it and rubbed it and then I rubbed it harder and harder with both hands and then he came. His cum just jumped out of the end of it, beautiful big white blobs. One of them went so high that it landed on my shoulder and dripped down my back. The rest of them I smeared all over my breasts, pulling my nipples and squeezing myself.

"After that we lay side by side for over half an hour, almost completely silent, all sticky with syrup and cunt juice and cum. We didn't say much but then we didn't need to say much because we had found ourselves again, and I had found my self-confidence, and I knew now that everything between us was going to be all right, no matter what problems we had."

Kylie, 27, who jointly managed an equestrian center near Butte, Montana, with her partner, Jim, found that the rigors of the job were having a serious effect on their love life. "Jim always came to bed too tired, too worried about money, too concerned about the horses. He didn't seem to have any time for me at all, except as somebody to share his problems and to lighten his workload. We hardly ever made love and when we did he was very distracted, like he was thinking about bridles and bits instead of how to give me an orgasm.

"I tried to talk to him about it. We'd always been able to discuss just about everything, but this time I couldn't seem to make any progress. He nodded and said, 'Sure,' and admitted that he hadn't been paying me enough mind, but that was as far as it went. It didn't change anything. We were always up very early in the morning and we didn't have time to make love before breakfast, which has always been my favorite time; and in the evening it was the same old story. Too tired, too stressed out. The weekends? Well, they were worse, if anything, because the weekend was always our busiest time.

"Worst of all, I began to realize that Jim never really *noticed* me any more. He didn't notice what I wore, he never said that he liked my hair, the way he used to. Don't get me wrong. He was still very affectionate and I didn't have any fears that he was seeing another woman. I guess he just needed me to catch his one-hundred-percent attention and say, 'Look at me! Remember me? I'm the girl you couldn't get enough of! Now you don't seem to be interested in me at all!"

Kylie wasn't attracted to the idea of wearing erotic underwear. "I just don't think it's me . . . I'm too much of an outdoors girl, you know? I couldn't pretend to be a lady of the night. And I'm not too sure how Jim would react. He used to like these little white lace panties I wore. He said they made me look like a virgin and that really turned him on. So I wasn't at all sure that if I looked like a girl who definitely *wasn't* a virgin . . . in a peephole bra, you know, and a sequined G-string, that he'd appreciate that.

"Another thing about him, in spite of the fact that our love life has been falling apart, he's still very possessive. He doesn't like other men looking at me and if a man pays me a compliment he puts on this face like he's going to punch the other guy out. He never used to be like that before."

I talked to Jim, and his possessiveness gave me a clear indication of his state of mind. He was stressed about his business because, although it was reasonably successful, it was much harder work than he had imagined and it wasn't showing the immediate returns that he had expected. He had always promised Kylie that he would give her a life of luxury. But the simple truth was that he had been overly optimistic and couldn't deliver. So on top of his other problems—mortgage, bank loans, veterinary bills, and the day-to-day running of the equestrian center—he felt that he had let Kylie down, and he was worried that she wouldn't want to stay with him if he didn't give her the lifestyle that he had promised her.

In reality he had nothing to fear because Kylie was very much in love with him and was prepared to stay with him even if the center went bankrupt. But Jim's confidence in himself had taken a severe blow and that had also diminished his sexual self-confidence. He was beginning to avoid making love to Kylie because he was afraid that he might let her down in bed, too.

He was behaving more possessively because he was afraid that his apparent lack of sexual interest in her would eventually lead her to look for satisfaction with somebody else.

This was the point where Kylie needed to take control of their love life, restore Jim's confidence, and find satisfaction where she really wanted to find it—with him. Since Jim's sexual tastes seemed to lean toward the simple and the virginal, and he would probably be put off by Kylie dressing as "a lady of the night," as she put it, I suggested that she wear simple, everyday clothes, but in a very erotic way.

The first thing she did was to shave off all of her pubic hair. "I like my cunt like that . . . it looks very fresh and untouched, but at the same time you can see everything. I only have to open my legs a little way and you can see all of my cunt lips and clitoris and right up inside my vagina. It's young and innocent, but at the same time it's very provocative, isn't it, because you're showing your lover everything you've got.

"On Wednesday morning, when Jim came back from taking the horses out, I was having breakfast. I was wearing a big oatmeal-colored sweater and sloppy socks, but that was all. Jim sat down and helped himself to a cup of coffee, and I went to the sink to clear up the dishes. All of a sudden Jim said, 'Are you wearing any panties?' and I could feel my heart bump. I didn't know how he was going to react at all. I said, 'No, why?' He said, 'You wouldn't want to catch cold, would you?' and at first I thought I hadn't succeeded in turning him on at all. But he stood up and he put his arms around me, and he slid his hand up inside my sweater at the back and he caressed the cheeks of my butt. He kissed me, and he said, 'I think you look cute. In fact, I think you look more than cute. You look like a million dollars. And a million dollars is just what I need right now.'

"He kissed me again, and squeezed my butt. Then he slid his hand farther up and felt my breasts, and he said, 'You're not wearing a bra, either.' I could feel his cock stiffening up through his jeans. I said, 'I decided that underwear isn't necessary when the best-looking man in Montana is around.' He played with my nipples and they crinkled up hard. Then he trailed his fingers down my side and around my waist and it gave me that great sexy tickling sensation. But it was when his fingers reached my cunt that he really flipped. He felt my hairless cunt-lips and he didn't say anything but he stared me right in the eyes and there was this look on his face like excitement, you know, and *wonder*, almost, if I can call it that. It was like a boy getting exactly what he had always wanted for Christmas.

"He stroked my cunt and then he opened it slightly and slid his finger inside. I was very excited myself by then, so it was easy. He took his finger out and sucked it, and he said, 'I haven't tasted anything as good as that in far too long.' He picked me up—he actually picked me up, just like I was a new bride—and he carried me into the bedroom. He striped off all of his clothes, but he didn't take off my sweater or my socks. He climbed onto the bed and he was beautiful looking. Dark hairy chest, muscular stomach, thighs like trees. A great forest of shaggy black pubic hair and this enormous cock sticking right up out of it with its big purple head and its great big hairy balls.

"He didn't say a word, but I could read everything I wanted to know in his face. He knelt between my legs and he gently opened up my cunt with his thumbs. Then he pushed his cock slowly into me, until his pubic hair was right up against my bare cunt lips, and it almost looked as if *his* pubic hair was mine.

"He fucked me slow, like he didn't want it ever to end. He kept on giving me these little kisses on my lips, over and over, and he looked into my eyes like he was seeing me for the very first time. I think he said something like 'You're unbelievable,' but we didn't say anything much. It was the joy of rediscovering just how good sex between us could be. We'd forgotten, you know, and I do think that people forget, especially when they've been together for quite a long time.

"First of all he fucked me on top. Then he changed position and lay beside me, so that he could play with my clitoris with his finger. I could reach down, too, and fondle his balls. They were so heavy and slippery with cunt juice, and I imagined that they must be full to bursting with sperm, all ready to shoot up inside me.

"He stroked my clitoris so light and gentle that I didn't realize that he was bringing me up to an orgasm. It just suddenly swelled up, do you know what I mean? And then there was nothing in the world but his huge cock up inside me, and his balls swinging against me, and his pubic hair all scrunched up against cunt lips. I could feel his cock inside me, I could feel every vein that was bulging out of it. It was like I was hyper-sensitive. And then I went into my orgasm, I couldn't stop myself any longer, and I was jumping and shouting but Jim held me tight so that all the time my cunt was going into spasm after spasm his cock was rammed right up inside me, enormously hard, and I couldn't get away from it.

"I thought he was ready to come, too, but while I was still twitching he took himself out of me and turned me over. He hadn't acted so strong and confident in bed for such a long time. He hadn't shown me how much he needed me. He pressed the head of his cock against my asshole, and pushed a little, not too hard, to show me that he wanted in.

"We had never done this before, and I wasn't at all sure about it. But Jim said, 'Come on, baby,' and pushed his cock against my asshole even harder. At first my asshole squinched up tight, and I don't think that he could have gotten a cotton-bud up it, let alone a full-size cock. But then he reached under my sweater and started to massage my breasts, rolling my nipples between his fingers, and I don't know, I just opened myself up to him, you know, and that enormous cock sank right into my ass, stretching my asshole so wide, until I could feel his pubic hair right up against me, yet again. It hurt. I can't say that it didn't. But it was a pain that you could die for, having your virgin asshole ravaged by the man you love, taking his cock deep and then taking it even deeper. I reached around and stroked his balls, and then I clawed them with my fingernails. Then I ran my fingers around my stretched-open asshole, and it was so sensitive, it was almost more sensitive than my clitoris. His cock slid in and out of me, and it was incredible. It was like going to the bathroom again and again—you know those times when you really need to go, and when it comes out it's such a pleasure that it's almost sexual. In the end he got harder and harder, and he started fucking me quicker and quicker. Then he suddenly grabbed hold of my shoulders and I could feel his cock pumping. He was coming, and he was shooting all of that beautiful baby-gravy right up inside my ass.

"When he took his cock out of me, I touched my asshole and it was stretched and sore and wide open. Jim opened up my legs and said, 'Look at that . . . you've lost your virginity.' And he licked my asshole very gently until it began to feel better. If you want to know what heaven's like, lie on a bed after a huge orgasm and have a man with designer stubble use his tongue to soothe your swollen asshole . . . that's heaven.

"That day was the beginning of our new love life. Even if we didn't make love every single day, because one or other of us was too tired, we still managed to make it three or four times a week, and each time it was better than the last. You wouldn't have thought that it was possible for a woman to save a terminal love life just by shaving her cunt and walking around with no panties on, but I did it, and it's lasted, and it's great."

Kylie managed to solve most of her problems because she was sensitive to Jim's sexual predilections. Obviously he wasn't aroused by stockings and garter belts and thongs. So she presented herself as the girl of his dreams. Innocent, young looking, with nothing on but socks and a sweater, unselfconsciously showing her freshly hairless vulva whenever she moved.

As sex commentator Leanne Owen put it, "I shave my pubes. Everyone who knows this generally hidden fact asks me the same questions. Does it make you look or feel sexier? Does it make you more sexually responsive? Does it turn your partner on? Well, let me tell you straight—yes, yes, and yes!"

Ms. Owen adds, "Shorn genitals, exposed and on show, no longer shielded by pubic hair, represents a peeling away of the final veil and symbolizes an unequivocal declaration of sexuality. Revealing your private parts in this way equals sex in the raw. The truth is that if you look sexy, you feel sexy and you want to have sex.

"But it is how my exposed pussy feels that is the clincher for me. It not only looks vulnerable, laid bare, womanly, but it's so much more tactile. With hairless genitals, there is a heightened awareness with every touch."

Kylie created an arousing erotic image of almost-accidental sexual exposure. She wasn't waiting on the couch when Jim came back from exercising his horses, dressed in a scarlet basque. Many men would have responded to that, but because of the deterioration of their relationship and the fact that Kylie had never worn anything like that before, Jim would have taken it as a sexual put-down. "You're so inadequate I have to dress up like this to save our sex life." In her sweater and her socks she was dressed as she normally would have done, but the surprise was the lack of panties—and then, the delayed surprise, the lack of pubic hair. Without having to say a single word, she was clearly telling him that she still wanted him, that he still turned her on, and that it was time for him to stop worrying so much about the business and start concerning himself with improving their love life.

You will have noticed how quickly Kylie's action restored Jim's sexual confidence. All he needed was to be reassured that she still wanted to tempt him and flirt with him, that he was still sexually attractive. The effectiveness of what she did can be judged by the fact that he treated her to anal intercourse, which is something that they had never tried before. Even though Kylie was the one who had taken control of their sexual relationship, she still had the pleasure of being "forcibly taken," which she found a very arousing experience indeed. So you can see that taking control of your love life and being (at times) a sexually submissive partner are not necessarily incompatible.

"I loved it taking his cock up my ass," she said afterward. "I closed my eyes while he was doing it, and I thought to myself, this is wonderful. Now he's had me in every hole. We've done it again since, but nothing could ever beat that first time."

It takes only a little imagination to dress yourself to thrill. Helen, 23, a magazine journalist from New York, told me that she stimulates her husband, Paul, on weekends by walking around all day in various degrees of nudity. "Sometimes I'll wear nothing all day but a pair of shoes; or a pair of panties; or a hat. Then we'll go out in the evening and I won't tell him whether I'm wearing any panties or not—not until we arrive at the dinner party or the theater or wherever we're going. I remember we went to a concert at Carnegie Hall, and when the orchestra was tuning up, I bent over to Paul and said, 'It's all right . . . I'm wearing panties tonight.' He said, 'Okay, fine.' And then I said, 'You wait till you see them.' He said, 'Why?' and he kept on asking me what they were like, right up until the first interval. Then I said, 'They're shiny black latex.' He said, *'Wow,'* which I kind of knew that he would, because he thinks that rubber is very sexy. He bought me a rubber miniskirt once but I never wore it. I guess I should have, even if I didn't strut around in it outside the house. Anyhow, I said, 'Not only are they shiny black latex, they have double dildoes inside them. Two solid black rubber dildoes, one up my cunt and the other up my ass.'

"You should have seen his face! He would have left the concert right there and then and taken me to the nearest hotel. But in the end he calmed down and we listened to the end of the concert.

"When we got back home, though, he practically tore my dress off. And, no, I wasn't telling lies. I was actually wearing black rubber panties with dildoes inside them. I had been researching an article on fetish fashion and a mail-order company had sent me a sample pair. I tried them, and I adored them. They were kind of clammy to start with, but once they warm up to your body temperature, you soon get used to them. And those dildoes! Every time you stand up or sit down or walk to the elevator, you're double-fucking yourself. I didn't quite have an orgasm, but there were two or three moments when I thought that I was close.

"Paul slowly rolled my panties off. They made a squeaky, rubbery, snapping sound, and they smelled strong, too—not just latex but the smell of cunt. I think Paul got a hell of a thrill out of seeing that big black rubber cock sliding out of my vagina, and then the thinner cock coming out of my anus, *schloop*!

"When my panties were off, Paul turned them inside-out and sucked both rubber cocks, and while he did so, his own cock came up as if it was on a string. I said, 'You shouldn't lick that . . . it's been up my ass all evening.' He said, 'All the more reason. And these taste so much like you . . . now I want to taste the real you.' He climbed onto the bed and he made love to me like he'd never made love to me before. He kissed me all over, he even sucked my toes and kissed my feet. He fucked me beautifully—one of those strong rhythmic fucks with both of us going in perfect synchronicity, I call it 'Swing Low, Sweet Chariot' fucking.

"When he was about to come, he took himself out of me, and knelt astride me on the bed. He started to masturbate himself but I wouldn't let him. As far as I was concerned, that was *my* job!

"I took hold of his cock and rubbed it, and it didn't take more than four or five rubs before he shot sperm all over my face and into my hair, and over my breasts, too. He held me close for over twenty minutes, and in any case I didn't want to move. I lay there with sperm dripping into my ears and sperm clinging in my eyelashes, and I felt as if I'd been anointed."

Even if you're not dressing specifically to be sexy, it's always worth taking extra trouble with your clothes and your appearance. It's a compliment to your partner, a way of showing him that you think he's the best. Don't overdo it, however. It's possible to wear too much in the way of facial cosmetics while trying for a look of absolute perfection—hair, teeth, nails, trim figure, etc.—whereas some of the sexiest women are the women who look well groomed but *accessible.* Nothing deters a man more than a woman in a power suit with clawlike nails, highly polished shoes and a flawless *coiffure* that's a masterpiece in solidified hairspray.

Think of some of the memorably sexy images from the movies—Brigitte Bardot with her blouse knotted, Sophia Loren with her dress torn halfway across her breast, Raquel Welch in her mammoth-skin bikini, Kate Winslet in her wet dress as the *Titanic* goes down—and you can see that dressing to thrill is not just about clothes but about the way you use those clothes to emphasize your most attractive features and your sexual personality . . . to focus your partner's attention on what it is about you that's sexy and stimulating.

Wash the car in a white blouse, making sure that you splash yourself so that your nipples show through. Do your household chores in nothing but a crop-top sweater and a lace thong. Pick your partner up from the station in a severe black turtleneck and black high heels and nothing else. Go to the market in winter in a heavy overcoat and a wool hat and gloves, but remain naked underneath and make sure that your partner knows it (although you should watch out for those in-store video cameras, unless you want to start a career in porn videos!)

Above all, don't let your partner forget that you're a sexy-looking woman with a strong sexual appetite and that you're looking to him for satisfaction. You want really great sex and you have to galvanize him into giving it to you.

Hair, makeup, and jewelry come under the heading of "dressing to thrill," too. If you've had the same hairstyle since leaving high school, maybe it's time you went to your hairdresser for something more startling. Change your color or change your cut. I talked to literally scores of men about what clothes and hairstyles they found the sexiest, and over 60 percent said they were aroused by very short spiky crops or short hair slicked back with gel. Thirty percent said that they liked long blonde hair, but the impression frequently created by girls with very long hair or elaborate hairstyles was that they were more interested in their own appearance than they were in giving a man a good time. Dan, 23, from Madison, Wisconsin, told me, "I once went out with a very pretty girl whose blonde hair was so long she could sit on it. But it was like going out with two people instead of one—her and her hair. It was always 'Watch my hair!' or 'Your watchstrap's caught in my hair' or 'I can't go out tonight . . . it's raining and my hair will get wet.' "

Definite turn-offs for most men are French braids ("librarian . . . schoolmarm . . . sexually repressed") and any kind of Trapp-family braids. They like natural and wild, or short and severe. Roger, 33, a psychiatrist from Boston, Massachusetts, told me, "A woman with very short hair looks as if she's in charge, but at the same time she also looks vulnerable. Women use their hair to hide themselves. A woman with very short hair is saying, 'Look at me. I'm naked. I'm hiding nothing. This is the way I am.' It's scary, but at the same time it's highly erotic."

This is what "dressing to thrill" is all about. Creating an erotic tension by contrasting clothed with naked, bare skin with fabric, modesty with blatancy. And it certainly doesn't require an enormous outlay, even if you do decide to spend a couple of hundred dollars on open-crotch panties and bras with heart-shaped holes for your nipples to poke through.

You could dress to thrill in something as plain and simple as a T-shirt. Two sisters from San Diego, California, told me in a long letter how they had aroused the men in their lives by holding their own wet T-shirt contest—with a difference, as you will see! Sara, 27, is a ceramic artist, and her sister, Laurene, 24, is currently unemployed, but has lived for nearly a year with Sara and her husband, Jeff, a kitchen installer.

I wasn't entirely sure how much of Sara's story was true and how much of it was fantasy. Normally I don't include personal anecdotes unless I can be sure that they are all or mostly true. (I'm tolerant about a little exaggeration now and again.) But I talked to Sara on the telephone for a long time and it was obvious that she and her sister were both very highly sexed, though occasionally she would go off on a long erotic story that sounded as if it were wishful thinking rather than something that had actually happened. But after I had talked to Laurene, too, it became clear that in spite of their sexually active imaginations they had very distinct ideas about what they wanted from their sexual relationships and what they wanted from their men. They had grasped the essential secret of really great sex, which is taking control.

The wet T-shirt contest story I believe to be substantially true, but even if the following account rings hollow to you, it still shows how you can give the man if your life a truly memorable sexual experience by the way you dress.

"Laurene has been living with me and Jeff ever since she split up from her boyfriend Bobby. Bobby was a great guy but he was a musician and he was always on the road, which meant that he was always cheating on her, and she couldn't take it anymore. We live close to Balboa Park. We have a very pretty apartment with a brick backyard. It's real small but that doesn't really matter because Laurene and I have always gotten along real good and there's never any friction between us. Well—some sexual friction. When we were younger we used to lie in bed together at night and wonder what it would be like to make love to a man, and we'd kiss each other's breasts, pretending we were men, and sometimes we'd masturbate each other. The first person to give me an orgasm was my sister, Laurene. When we started dating, we shared the same boyfriend a couple of times. I mean we'd both go out with him and we'd both go to bed with him, both at the same time.

A threesome, that's it. We both had the same taste in boys . . . moody-looking guys with curly hair and blue eyes and stubble. So instead of one of us getting jealous, we shared, and usually the guy couldn't believe his luck.

"That's how Laurene and I taught ourselves to make love to a man, both of us together. We would kiss him both at once, so that he had two tongues struggling to get into his mouth. Then we would fondle him all over, and scratch him a little, and bite his nipples, things like that. It drove them totally crazy, especially when Laurene went down and started to suck his cock, and then I would sit right over his face and hold my pussy wide open so that he could lick it. Sometimes the two of us would suck his cock together, and have tongue fights. We'd lick him all the way down the shaft of his cock, one of us on each side, and you should have heard him groan! Then Laurene would take one ball right in her mouth and I would take the other, and we'd bite and tug and see how much pain the poor guy could take. We'd take it in turns to fuck him, and while I was riding up and down on him, for instance, Laurene would fondle the guy's balls with one hand and diddle my clitoris with the other, so that I got so aroused that I was practically out of my head.

"Even when the guy had climaxed, we soon got him hard again by putting on a show—kissing each other and fondling each other's breasts and making all the right panting noises. Laurene was always more into this than I was. Laurene loved to lick my pussy . . . she was always doing it, even when we didn't have a boy there. Sometimes I used to wake up in the middle of the night and Laurene would have my legs wide open and be licking me, right up inside me, with a finger up my asshole. I liked it. I can't say that I didn't. But she was my sister, and I never felt that it was right. I did it once or twice, just flicking her clitoris with the tip of my tongue, but she liked to go the whole way, you know, rubbing her face right into my wet pussy, and going 'Mmm-mmm! Slurp! Slurp!' sucking every last drop out of me when I came. She isn't a lesbian. She's not interested in other women, as far as I know. She loves me, that's all, and she loves sex, and I guess she felt that was a way in which she could please me and turn herself on at the same time.

"Jeff liked having her around at first. I mean, what man wouldn't? She has long brunette hair and a fabulous figure, thirty-six DD and a waist you could close your hands around, and the longest legs. But after a while I began to think that he missed the privacy we used to have. He's the kind of guy who likes to come home and sit in front of the TV for a while before he'll even tell you what his day was like. He likes to have his friends around, too, and they'll all drink beer and watch baseball and that's when I usually go to my studio and do some painting on my own. But Laurene isn't a girl for going into hiding when there are guys around, especially now that she doesn't have a regular guy of her own. So whenever Jeff brought his friends over she was always flirting with them, sitting on their knees and teasing them by snatching away their cans of beer. They were quite cute guys but I don't think they had the nerve to come on to her, you know, especially since she was Jeff's sister-in-law.

"One afternoon we were sitting outside in the yard having a drink and the guys were inside watching the game, and they'd been inside for *hours*. Laurene said, 'I'm really bored with this and I'm really frustrated. How can we get those guys to fuck us?' At first I couldn't believe what she was saying, but she was serious. She said, 'You can fuck Jeff and I'll fuck the other two. It'll be great. You know, like an orgy.'

"Before I could stop her she went into the den and said, 'Hey guys, why don't you stop watching that stupid baseball and give us a good time?' They didn't believe her, either, they thought she was teasing again. So she came back outside and said, 'Don't worry . . . I'll get them going. We'll have a wet T-shirt contest, just you and me.' By this time I was kind of entering into the spirit of it, you know. We'd drunk over a bottle and a half of wine between us and we were both feeling mischievous. We took off our jeans and Laurene took off her panties, too, these little filmy white lace things. Then we took off our bras and slipped them out through our sleeves. I said, 'I'll turn on the hose,' but Laurene said, 'Don't. I have a much better idea.' She went back to the door of the family room swinging her panties around her finger and said, 'Come on, guys, it's wet T-shirt time.'

"Well, this time they *did* believe her, and they came out into the yard carrying their cans of beer, Jeff and these two guys, Rick and Matthew. They were nice guys, good looking, and Matthew had this very curly hair that I adore. Laurene thought he looked like a saint.

"Jeff said to me, 'You're not going to show yourself in front of these guys, are you?' but I kissed him and said, 'Why not? It's only a game. And besides, I love you.'

"Matthew said, 'If this is a wet T-shirt contest, how come your T-shirts are dry?' But Laurene said, 'They won't be for long. But you don't think that *we're* going to do all the hard work, do you?' She knelt down in front of him and unbuckled his belt. Then she pulled open his buttons, and reached inside his jeans. He wasn't wearing shorts, and his cock came out, and it was stiffening up already. Laurene smiled at him and kissed his cock and rubbed it once or twice, but then she said, 'I don't want to make it *too* hard, do I, because then you won't be able to wet my T-shirt for me.' That was when the guys realized for the first time what she was talking about, and up until then, I have to say that I hadn't realized what she was talking about, either. Maybe some other time I would have thought it was disgusting, but right then, on that warm afternoon, with those three great-looking guys, and after all that wine, the idea of it gave me such a rush.

"I said, 'Come on, Jeff, let's show them how it's done.' I opened his pants and took out his cock. It wasn't hard yet, which was good, because it's almost impossible for a guy to piss when he's hard. Jeff said, 'You're serious? You really want to do it?' and all I did was lick my lips at him.

"Next to us, Matthew had suddenly started to piss on Laurene's T-shirt. A clear glittering stream that he played all over her breasts. Rick took out his cock and started to piss on her breasts, too. Her T-shirt clung to her body instantly, and you could see her nipples rising up underneath the wet cotton. Piss was running down her thighs and spattering onto the bricks. She crossed her arms and lifted her T-shirt up so that her breasts were bare, and the two of them stood right in front of her, Matthew and Rick, and hosed her body up and down so that she had piss running in streams from each stiff nipple.

"Right then, Jeff began to piss on me. It was a real gush, and I took hold of his cock and pulled it from side to side so that my T-shirt would be totally soaked. His piss was so fresh and warm that I lifted his cock so that he was spraying my face. I had my eyes and my mouth tight shut, but then I opened my lips so that he was pissing against my teeth, and then I opened my teeth, too, and my whole mouth was flooded. I swallowed three or four times, and it was delicious, but most of it ran down my chin.

"I opened my eyes and they stung a little. I looked across at Laurene and she was in her element. She was lying back on the sunbed now with her legs wide apart. She had Rick's cock in one hand and Matthew's in the other and she was directing their piss onto her clitoris and into her pussy.

"Jeff had finished now. He lifted me up and held me close and gave me a deep, piss-flavored kiss. He said, 'You and your sister . . . you've put me off baseball for life.' He stripped off his shirt and his pants, and he laid me down on the sunbed next to Laurene's. Rick and Matthew had finished, too, but Laurene was still licking Matthew's cock as if she couldn't get enough of him.

"Rick said, 'So what about the wet T-shirt contest?' and Jeff said, 'It's a draw. We'll have to arrange a replay.' Then right in front of everybody, totally unembarrassed, he pulled my panties to one side and slid his cock into my pussy. I never would have believed that he had confidence to do it, not in front of other guys. On the other hand I guess that Laurene and I had shown him that you can do absolutely anything if you want to, and it turns you on, and that includes pissing into your wife's mouth. I've pissed into *his* mouth since then, a couple of times, while he's been licking me, and the first time he climaxed without me even touching his cock.

"That afternoon went on for a long time . . . two or three hours. Rick and Matthew took turns to fuck Laurene. At one point she tried to get both of their cocks into her pussy at the same time, but they were too big for her, so Matthew fucked her in the ass instead. We all found that was such a turn-on. Her bright red asshole with this huge cock sliding in and out of it, her ass cheeks wobbling with every push, and the way she was crying out, 'Harder! Harder!' Toward the end she reached down between her legs and furiously masturbated herself, pulling and tugging at her pussy lips, her fingers really flying over her clitoris. She had an orgasm that almost doubled her up, and when she did, Matthew couldn't help climaxing, too.

"Some of the time Jeff and I watched and some of the time we went back to our own lovemaking. At the end of the afternoon we were all too tired to think about anything except taking a shower and crashing out.

"We haven't had another wet T-shirt contest since then and I don't think we ever will. I prefer it to stay like a memory, you know? Not so much a golden memory but a golden shower memory. It opened up a whole lot of new possibilities for me and Jeff. We're not afraid to discuss anything now, whether it's sexual or not. If I said, 'I want you to shit while you're making love to me so that I can feel it coming out of your ass,' he wouldn't be shocked. He'd probably say, 'Why not?' I believe that if two people love each other there is nothing that they can do together that's wrong or dirty. The only dirty thing about sex is the way some very repressed people think about it, and I feel sorry for them, because they don't know the pleasure they're missing."

Secret 5: Devote Yourself to His Delight

Women who learn to become generous sexual partners will almost always reap the reward of really great sex. I talk to so many women who are eager to improve their love lives—sometimes desperate for sexual satisfaction—yet who are still reluctant to take control of their relationships in order to get what they need and, yes, what they deserve.

Some women are inhibited by sheer timidity, especially women with partners who are sexually ignorant, or very straitlaced, or bullying, or insecure, or just plain pompous. "If I went down on him, he'd think that I was acting like some kind of hooker." "If I were to do anything fancy in bed, he'd be convinced that I'd found another man. No good trying to tell him that I learned it all from a book." "If I turned over in bed and started to feel his cock, he'd take that as criticism . . . like he wasn't keeping me satisfied and I had to come back to him for more."

Other women are wary because "I'm not very sexually experienced and I wouldn't really know what to do . . . supposing I made a fool of myself?"

Still more are plain resentful: "I always thought that when it came to sex it was a man's job to please the woman. Why should I do all the work?" "He never did anything creative and interesting to me. Why doesn't he stick his own finger up his ass? I'm not doing it."

But if your partner isn't giving you the really great sex that you deserve, you're going to have to face the fact that only one person can do something about it, and that's you. You have choices, of course. You may decide that you'd rather put up with the status quo than try to take control of your sex life. You may even decide that you would rather not bother and walk out of the relationship altogether: That's an option. It depends how much you think he's worth, and it depends on how much you think *you're* worth.

It's very important for you to understand this: Almost every dysfunctional sexual relationship is capable of being dramatically improved. It doesn't matter if we're talking about a relationship that is suffering severe psychological and/or physiological problems, such as frigidity or impotence, or a relationship that has run out of sexual tension because of financial stress or alcohol abuse, or even nothing more serious than over-familiarity and boredom. Even if you think your sexual relationship is "beyond saving," let me assure you that it isn't. I can't promise miracles. It may eventually turn out that you decide not to continue having sex with the same man. It may turn out that, if you're married, you want a divorce. But these are separate issues—issues for you to decide for yourself once you've discovered just how much better your sex life can be.

Throughout this book, I've been concentrating on showing you that sex isn't threatening or dirty or something that you can't openly discuss with your partner. As Sara said at the end of the previous chapter, no sexual activity between two people who love each other can be regarded as "wrong." What she and her sister Laurene did may be well beyond the limits of what some people find to be tasteful or acceptable. But everybody involved enjoyed it, everybody felt pleased and satisfied afterward, no laws were broken, nobody was hurt or distressed, and Sara's sexual relationship with Jeff was much improved. She drank a little of her husband's fresh urine, which is sterile, and which in limited quantities can actually prove to be beneficial to health. So what was "wrong" about that?

It isn't difficult to recognize the things that really *are* "wrong" in day-to-day sexual relationships. These are things that damage your relationship rather than cherish and improve it. Your sexual relationship is vital because it is the one arena where you and your partner don't have to put up any defenses—where you're both naked, body and soul, and you can put aside all of the stresses of the day and share each other's love. It's always tempting to use sex as a weapon, especially if you've had a blazing argument—"don't touch me!" But that's wrong, because it deprives you of a way in which you can use your mutual pleasure to work toward a reconciliation of ideas or, at the very least, a place where you can agree to disagree.

It's wrong for you to withhold sex from your partner just because you don't see eye-to-eye with him about something completely unrelated to your love life. It's equally wrong for your partner to expect you to be devoted to him if he can't or won't give you the sexual satisfaction you want.

It's wrong for you to lie to each other about sex. You can exaggerate your pleasure if you're really enjoying yourself, but don't fake orgasms and don't say that something turned you on if it didn't. It's wrong for your partner to bully you into sex or try to make you feel guilty if there's some sexual act that you really don't want to do. Most of all, it's wrong for either of you to take the other's sexual satisfaction for granted.

However, it can never be wrong for him to give you pleasure and excitement, no matter how he does it: with his cock, his fingers, his tongue, or an oversized vibrator. And whatever sexual fantasies he might be having while he's making love to you, they're not wrong, either. They might be very extreme. If he were to describe them to you in the cold light of day, they might sound totally filthy. But no sexual fantasy can be "wrong" in any meaningful sense. He might be fantasizing about sex on horseback with Xena the warrior princess while he's supposed to be making love to *you*. Why should that matter? Xena is just a mental stimulant, an aphrodisiac, whereas you're flesh and blood and warm and there in bed with him. He's not making love to her, he's making love to you, and if he's using her image to make you feel more stimulated, why should you worry? And ask yourself this: How many times have you lain underneath him while he worked his way toward a climax and wondered if you could remember that recipe for fried chicken? Is that worse than fantasizing about Xena?

I want to eliminate the words "dirty" and "wrong" from your sexual vocabulary. I want you to see all sexual activity as worth exploring, because, after all, there's a chance that you might find something that really transforms your love life forever. For instance, there's anal sex, which used to be regarded as a completely taboo subject. Yet these days, I have seen it freely and openly discussed by readers on the letters pages of magazines such as *Woman* and *Woman's Own*. I have had dozens of personal letters on the same subject, too.

"I feel amazing," said Lilian, 26, from Charleston, South Carolina. "I was frightened at first, but I took all of the precautions you mentioned in your book . . . lots of lubricant, pushing myself against him rather than squeezing myself tight. What can I say? I was ecstatic! I fucked him until he begged me to stop. I feel like I have two pussies now, instead of just one. I can take my husband in either, with equal ease and equal enjoyment. And he thinks I'm the most amazing woman that ever was."

Since first broaching the subject of wet sex more than ten years ago, I have received more letters and calls on that single subject than almost any other, from women in particular, who felt liberated when I encouraged them to enjoy the sensation. Do it standing up, do it in the shower. Do it anyplace you feel like it. As I said all those years ago, you don't have to feel embarrassed or repressed about openly pissing. You can use it as part of your lovemaking. As sex commentator Tuppy Owens remarked, "Many women are afraid of wetting the bed as they approach orgasm. What a shame that this fear prevents thousands of women from reaching a climax, when they should really just invest in a towel and enjoy!"

She added, "You can piss on each other at home in the bath or in the shower, but it's nice to do it on a hot day in the countryside, preferably next to a river, stream, or waterfall where you can wash afterward. If you can't find a place to strip down and 'go the whole hog,' you can always put your hand in the stream while your lover is pissing up against a wall."

Only a few years ago, subjects like these were

hardly ever discussed outside of medical journals. But more and more people have come to understand that we're not talking about acts of violence or aggression here: We're talking about acts of *love*. We're talking about ways to make our sexual partners feel pampered and wanted and sexually stimulated.

You can use those techniques to make your partner feel really, really good—better than a movie star. But before he arrives back home, it's worth picking up a paper and pad, and working out what you really want out of your sex life. List the pros on one side, cons on the other.

Do you want to continue in the same old way? Or are you prepared to take a risk and see if you can't change your sex life forever? How far are you prepared to go to excite your partner? Be honest now . . . if there are sexual acts that you really don't like the idea of, then don't force yourself. Just be aware that they exist, and don't totally condemn them out of hand. Some people enjoy them, even if you don't think that you would.

One of the reasons I gave you a list of porn videos earlier in this book was not so much to assess your preferences, or even to think about what turns you on and what doesn't, but for you to judge for yourself how shockable you are—or maybe how adventurous you're prepared to be. Although some of the videos may have sounded very extreme, none of them catered toward anything more than what you might call standard run-of-the-mill sexual fantasies.

They featured the usual suspects: teenage girls, young Oriental girls, big-breasted women, group orgies, larger women, oral sex, anal sex, water sports, sub/dom, gays, and animals. They all sell very well, so somebody must be buying them, and they get thousands of repeat orders, too.

You can safely assume that *all* men have at least a passing curiosity in the kind of sexual activity that these videos depict. If your partner assures you that he doesn't, then he is either lying or he has already seen so many that he doesn't want to see any more. But don't assume that just because your partner is aroused by the sight of a woman giving sexual favors to five football players that he wants you to do the same. Videos like these are fuel for sexual fantasies, that's all. They offer vicarious pleasure, just like travel videos or cooking videos or action-adventure videos. Nobody thinks it's degrading to sit in front of a TV screen and salivate while Ken Hom stir-fries a Chinese chow mein, so where is the logic in saying that it is degrading to be aroused by pictures of people making love? Many single people use porn videos as an aid to masturbation, while many couples find that watching a porn video while they are in bed together helps to prolong and intensify their lovemaking.

Discussing sexual fantasies can do an enormous amount to renew the closeness of your sexual relationship, but here again you will probably have to make the first move. Although they may watch porn videos and look at men's magazines, most men are embarrassed to admit it. Sometimes the very secrecy of it is part of the thrill. It gives them a feeling of doing something "forbidden," and that feeling can be a very potent part of what makes sex exciting.

When they discover that their husbands or partners are reading or watching pornography, many women feel extremely threatened and confused. Pat, 37, from Pittsburgh, Pennsylvania, said, "I found some videotapes in my husband's desk. I'd needed some blank tapes so I played them to make sure that there was nothing on them we wanted to keep. I've never been so horrified in my life. They were full of young girls sucking men's penises and letting them climax all over their faces. I didn't know what to think. I felt as if in all these years of marriage, I hadn't been enough to keep Stanley happy. I felt plain and sexless and completely inadequate."

I reassured Pat that if her husband was still with her and their love life was reasonably active then there was nothing for her to worry about. In fact the discovery of her husband's videos gave her a unique opportunity to improve their lovemaking.

"When Stanley came back from his business trip, I gave him a drink, relaxed him, and started making supper. It wasn't easy, telling him that I had found his videos. I'm not the kind of person who can just come out and say, 'Ah-ha! You'll never guess what happened today! I was poking around in your desk and I came across these utterly disgusting videos!

They're not yours, of course?' No—what I *did* say was, 'I was looking for some blank videotapes and I found these in your desk. And I checked to see what was on them. And I apologize for invading your privacy. But I'm not shocked'—that was a little bit of a lie—'and I really don't mind at all.' that was another little bit of a lie. 'And I was wondering if maybe we could watch them together so that I could see what kinds of things turn you on."

I had cautioned Pat to take things very, very easy when she first told Stanley about her discovery. Stanley was going to feel embarrassed and guilty and maybe angry, too. The important thing was to reassure him that she didn't think any less of him, and that she considered it perfectly normal for him to have porn videos in his desk (which, of course, it was). All she had to introduce was a slight note of resentment that he hadn't shared his interest with her. "He muttered something like, 'I didn't think you'd like them.' So I said, 'I won't know until I've seen them properly, will I?' "

By showing curiosity rather than resentment, Pat was able to help Stanley to overcome his embarrassment, and by the time they had finished supper that evening, he was positively enthusiastic about showing them to her. "I was extremely nervous but I tried not to show it. Imagine being nervous with your own husband! But it was like I was seeing a new side to him that he had never shown me before. You know, the dark side of the moon. I always thought that we had a very good sex life. We used to make love two or three times a week, sometimes more often. When I look back on it now, it wasn't very *varied* lovemaking. Once the children were away for the weekend and we made love on the couch while we listened to all of our old songs, 'This Time the Girl Is Going to Stay,' romantic things like that. But mostly we made love in bed the way that normal people do. I didn't really go for oral sex, either. Stanley tried to do it to me every now and then but I was never very comfortable. I suppose that was partly because I felt that if I let him do it to me, he'd expect me to do it to him, and, to be frank, I didn't have any idea what to do. I asked my closest friend Francine about it once but all she said was, 'You can't *tell* anybody how to do it! You just *do* it!' and that wasn't very helpful.

"We showered and got ourselves ready for bed. I thought of putting on one of my sexy satin nighties but then I thought that would look as if I was expecting to get turned on and what if I wasn't? What if it turned out be dreadful and I couldn't stand it? But Stanley came in with two glasses of champagne, and I thought, I hope this turns out to be a celebration and not a row."

I had previously explained to Pat what she might expect to see in her husband's videos. She wasn't so naïve that she had no idea about pornography at all, but she had never seen any, neither had she ever felt the urge to see any, and her own sex life was so straightforwarrd that she had only a superficial knowledge about different sexual positions, about oral or anal sex, or variations such as spanking or bondage or rubberwear. "There are things that you hear about, aren't there, and you know that they happen, but you don't necessarily want to hear all the intimate details."

However, I advised her to keep an open mind and see if she couldn't try to enjoy what she was about to see. Stanley had bought the videos not because he didn't love her, or didn't find her sexually attractive any longer. He had bought them to bring a little erotic variety into his life and to stoke up his fantasies. Maybe she could join in those fantasies, and make them even more stimulating for him.

"In the first scene, two young men were walking along a beautiful white sandy beach. They saw a blonde girl sitting by the dunes. She was wearing a very small blue bikini. She was pretty, and her breasts were enormous. They scarcely fitted into her bikini top, and she was showing the edges of her nipples. Actually I thought that was quite sexy. I used to have a summer dress when I was in college that was so low-scooped that I had to keep tugging it up so that it wouldn't show my nipples, and I remember how sexy I used to feel in that. All the guys would be trying to look me in the eye when they talked to me but their eyes always kept straying down to my breasts.

"I guess you could say that was my first turning-point while looking at this video. I remembered how sexy I used to be when I was younger, and I suddenly thought: What's happened to me? Where's that feeling of being completely free, of letting myself go, of being myself? Here's this young girl smiling and chatting with these young men, and *I* used to be like that.

"The girl knelt upon the sand and she started to fondle one of the young men's swimshorts. You could see that he had an erection. She pulled his shorts down and his penis was sticking up hard. I hadn't seen another man's penis since I married Stanley, not that close. The video was so sharp that you could see every vein. What amazed me was that he was completely shaved, no pubic hair at all. I know that women do it. I trim my own pubic hair with nail scissors. But I didn't know that men did it, and it looked—I don't know, it looked bigger than Stanley's, and very smooth, as if you wanted to run your hand along it, as if you wanted to—"

Lick it?

"Yes, I suppose you're right. It looked like something you'd like to lick. Especially the top of it, which was very purple and shiny; and the testicles, which were very tight and wrinkled up, but no hair at all!"

So then what happened?

"The girl pulled down her bikini top so that her breasts spilled out of it. She lifted her hands and squeezed her breasts together to give herself a really tight cleavage. The young man took his penis in his hand and pushed it between her breasts as if he was making love to her vagina. I couldn't believe how clear the pictures were, how close up. He stood over this girl and made love to her breasts as if he was making love to her vagina. Then before he could climax, she stopped squeezing her breasts so tight together, and she took hold of his penis and started to lick it. At first her tongue just danced around the tip, although now and then she let it dart into his hole, as quick as a snake. But then she stuck her tongue right out and licked his testicles, and all around the base of his penis, and then back to his testicles again. The video was so close that you could watch the tip of her tongue exploring every single wrinkle in his scrotum, and then diving down into the darkness to seek out his anus.

"I tried to imagine that I was watching a video of me and Stanley. I even wondered what it would be like if I shaved Stanley's penis. I touched Stanley's leg. Then I went a little farther and slid my hand into his open pajamas. He was hard already. I stroked his penis up and down and he put his arm around me and said, 'Pat . . .' and that was the first time I'd heard him say, 'Pat . . .' in that particular way for a long, long time. It sounded like 'Pat, I adore you . . . Pat, I'm passionate for you . . . Pat, I want to make love to you over and over.' But he didn't have to say any of that. I could hear it in the way he just said, 'Pat . . .'

"The girl in the video kissed the man's penis and

then she dug her teeth into it, not too hard, but deep enough for her lower teeth to sink right into his hole. She looked at the camera like a lioness that's caught her prey and is just *daring* you to take it away from her. But then she opened her mouth wider and took down the whole of his penis, deeper and deeper, and you could see her almost choking, but she kept on taking it farther and farther until his shaven balls were dangling on her chin.

"She didn't really suck so much as make love to him with her mouth, bobbing her head up and down and giving his penis amazing twirling licks with the end of her tongue. At the same time she was rubbing him up and down . . . I was surprised at how hard. I had tried rubbing Stanley's penis once, but after a while it had only seemed to make him irritable. I realized then that I hadn't been doing it nearly hard enough.

"While all this was going on, the second man had taken off his swimshorts and was standing close by, playing with himself. He had a big penis, too—very big and very red, I remember, with lots of blond pubic hair. The girl reached over with her free hand and started to rub him, too.

"Suddenly the first man took his penis out of her mouth. She gave it two or three more quick rubs and he shot cum all over her cheek. She opened her mouth really wide and stuck out her tongue and he shot more cum right onto her tongue. Some of it even squirted right down her throat. There was a close-up of all those sticky white drops on her tongue. Then, without putting her tongue back into her mouth, she turned to the other man, took hold of his penis, and wiped it on her tongue from side to side, so that it was smothered with the first man's cum. Then she started to suck him and lick him and roll her tongue around him.

"I was *very* turned on. The girl in the video was so beautiful, so classy. If you saw her at a party, say, fully dressed, I think it would be hard for you to guess what she did for a living. And she couldn't have been much older than twenty, or twenty-one. Still, she might have been young but she taught *me* what oral sex was all about.

"I drew back the bedcovers. Stanley's penis was very stiff and sticking out of his pajamas. He laid his hand on my shoulder and he was quite tense. For a moment I thought he was going to say, "Don't do it." But I kissed the top of his penis and then I licked it and then I took it into my mouth, and I felt him relax, as if this was something he had been waiting for, and at last it had happened.

"I tried to suck him and lick him in the same way that the girl in the video had been sucking and licking, although I tried a few flourishes of my own so that he wouldn't think I was just trying to copy her. For instance, I licked his testicles with the flat of my tongue and then I gave him a big broad lick all the way up his cock until I got to the top. I did that three or four times and he said, 'Oh, baby . . .' and ran his fingers through my hair. Then I pointed my tongue and pushed the very tip of it into the little hole in the top of his cock. While I was doing that I looked up and our eyes met. Stanley smiled at me and slowly shook his head to tell me that he couldn't believe that what was happening to him was true. The feeling of pleasure and excitement I got from his face was wonderful. And for the first time I had a feeling of *power*, too: a feeling that I could turn him on whenever I wanted to—whenever *I* felt like being satisfied, rather than having to wait for *him* to feel like it.

"The video was still going on, and I could hear a different girl moaning as two men were making love to her. I was aching to have Stanley's penis up inside me, and I was very tempted to climb on top of him. But now I knew that I could excite him anytime I felt like it, and I thought, let me try this first . . . then we'll make love later. I held his cock tight, so tight that my fingernails dug into it, and I rubbed it up and down so hard that the skin stretched. I licked and sucked the end of his penis, and did the same swirling thing with my tongue that the girl in the video had been doing.

"Stanley suddenly gripped me tight. I could feel that he was just about to come, so I took his penis out of my mouth and stuck out my tongue. The next thing I knew he was spraying warm cum all over my face. It was everywhere—sticking in my eyelashes, dripping down the side of my nose—but a lot of it was on my tongue, too. I gave Stanley's penis a few final rubs just to make sure that I had emptied him dry. He was beginning to go soft already. Then I moved up the bed. I had to curl my tongue to keep the cum from dropping off it. I kissed Stanley right on the lips, and slid my tongue into his mouth, and we kissed deeper and deeper, and shared the taste of his climax.

"We made love four times that night, which was a record for us. The second time I sucked Stanley's soft penis back into life; and the third time I was asleep, but Stanley woke me up by licking my vagina. I had two orgasms, and when I woke up in the morning I was tired but I was very, very happy; and I knew that things were going to be different from now on."

I am often surprised by the way in which oral sex (fellatio) is regarded in the United States. Feminists seem to think that it is a submissive act, simply because it sometimes involves a woman being on her knees in front of a man. Of course this is very rarely the case, unless the woman gives her partner a blow job someplace where it's impossible to lie down—such as in an office. It can be a considerable strain for the man to stand upright as his sexual tension increases, and it's very much easier for the woman to give him the full benefit of her tongue technique if he's lying down.

There is nothing at all submissive about fellatio. In fact it is the one sexual act in which a woman has complete control over her partner's sexual arousal. She can decide whether to do it, when to do it, and how to do it. She can stop halfway through, if she wants to, or she can go on until her partner reaches a climax. She can do it when he's soft and she can do it when he's hard. She can make it quick or she can make it very, very slow. And when he does eventually come, it is entirely up to her whether she swallows his semen, or decorates her face with it, or smears it on her breasts, or simply lets it fly every which way.

Fellatio can be used as foreplay or it can be a complete sexual act in itself. You can use it as a way of arousing your man's interest before you make love or if you don't feel like intercourse you can use it to keep him satisfied without having to go as far as full penetration. This is especially useful when you're pregnant or when you're having your period (although an increasing number of young women are continuing to have sex during their period and enjoying it . . . more on that later).

Jeanne, a 34-year-old receptionist from Houston, Texas, said that her whole marriage was dramatically improved when she started to give her husband, Douglas, oral sex at odd moments during the day and night. "I wouldn't say that there was anything wrong with our marriage, but we were married young and by the time we reached our thirties our sex life had gotten kind of routine, to say the least. We made love two or three times a week but always in bed, and Douglas would introduce it, you know, by saying, 'Let's have an early night, okay?' and going to take a shower, so that I knew what was going to happen just as sure as I knew that the sun was going to rise the next morning.

"I read in one of your books how a woman could give a man oral sex at any time . . . when he was reading a book or watching TV or anytime at all. It's just plucking up the nerve to do it. So on the weekend when Douglas had his feet up on the couch watching TV I brought in a fresh beer for the both of us. I knelt on the floor beside the couch and opened up his can for him, and opened mine, too, and said, 'Cheers.' I stayed there for a while just talking to him and then I let my hand stray down and touch him through his pants. He said, 'Hey, what're you doing?' but not annoyed or anything. I said, 'I'm just checking that it's still there,' and I stroked his cock through his pants until it began to stiffen up. He said, 'Is it still there?' and I said, 'I'd just better make sure,' and I tugged down his zipper and took his cock out of his pants. 'Well, it's still there,' I said. 'I'd better check that it still tastes as good.' And I pulled down his foreskin and gave him a long lick, like I was licking a Popsicle. His cock went really hard, and when I glanced at him to see what his reaction was, he had this expression on his face like, 'What's going on here? This is too good to be true.' I started to suck his cock good and deep, and all the time I kept my eyes on his. I made a real show of it—kissing and licking the end of his cock and rubbing it against my lips, and then rolling it against my face. Then I put it back in my mouth and gave him such a sucking, long and slow, and each time I sucked I went 'Mmmm' and made my whole body shiver like I was sucking him right down to my toes.

"He said, 'I can't take any more of this,' and he sat up, unbuckled his belt, and pulled off his pants faster than I ever saw him pull off his pants before, even when we first started having sex. He laid me down on the rug and lifted up my dress, and he tugged my panties to one side so that my pussy was exposed. He lifted my right leg and put it through the arm of the couch, and then he pulled one of the chairs across and lifted my left leg and put it through the arm of the chair, so that my legs were wide apart and I couldn't do anything about it. He leaned over me and he kissed me. He hadn't shaved and his chin was stubbly but I didn't mind at all. I ran my hands through his hair and I took hold of his ears so that he wouldn't stop kissing me and while he was kissing me he rubbed his cock up and down between the lips of my cunt and then he pushed it into me.

"I could hardly believe it. There we were, fucking on the floor in the middle of the afternoon, and me with my legs trapped. It was one of the greatest fucks we'd ever had. What was best of all was that I had an orgasm first—an incredible, shattering orgasm—and what made it all the more shattering was that I couldn't close my legs together like I usually do when I come, so for some reason that made it go on and on, lots of aftershocks and twitches. Douglas went on fucking me without even breaking his rhythm, and that started building me up toward another orgasm almost right away. I had that really strange feeling between my legs that I wanted him to go on fucking me but at the same time I wanted him to stop. I had another orgasm that wasn't quite an orgasm, it was more like a spasm, you know, when you're falling asleep and you jolt and you wake yourself up. But that was enough to make Douglas come. He kissed me and his tongue went down my throat so deep I thought he could almost lick the top of his cock, down there inside me. But just as he came he took his cock out and squirted his sperm all over my cunt lips and my panties.

"We lay there for a while, exhausted, and then he freed my legs and helped me up. He kissed me again and said, 'What did you do that for?' and I said, 'What?' and he said, 'Going down on me like that, for no reason.' And I said, 'There *was* a reason. I love you and I wanted to show you, and I didn't want to wait until bedtime.' He liked that. He liked that a lot. And he liked it when I took off my panties and held them up against my nose and said, 'That's you . . . that's the beautiful smell of you.'

"Now I give him oral sex wherever and whenever. I gave it to him when he was in the bathtub a couple of nights ago. I gave it to him when he was sitting at his desk, trying to work out his accounts. But the best time was when he was talking on the phone to his boss. I took out his cock and licked it until he forgot what he was trying to say and he had to tell his boss that there was somebody at the door and he'd better call him back.

"Demeaning? I don't think that giving a man oral sex is demeaning. It's not demeaning for a man to give a woman oral sex, is it? I do it when I feel like it, and not because Douglas wants it. Sometimes it ends up that we go the whole way, and sometimes it doesn't. All I can say is that it's made our sex life much less predictable and much more exciting."

You'll have noticed the lighthearted way in which Jeanne first initiated oral sex, treating it almost like a game. Lightheartedness is especially helpful if your partner is inhibited about sex at unusual times in unusual places. It will help to put him at ease, and make is seem far less obvious that you are taking control of your love life and having sex when *you* want it.

Oral sex can be varied enormously to give your partner a whole spectrum of exciting sensations. Apart from licking, sucking and (very) gentle biting, you can try changing the temperature inside of your mouth. In the Chinese sex manuals written before Ming times (circa 1500) it is recommended that a woman swallow hot green tea before taking her lover's penis into her mouth, so that his penis feels scalded; and the opposite effect can be achieved these days if you crunch some crushed ice in your mouth before you give your partner oral sex. You can add flavor to the experience with your favorite fruit syrup.

I have heard of many other unusual ways in which women have excited their partners during oral sex. One woman told me that she took a mouthful of spaghetti before she went down on her boyfriend, so that she could "swirl all that pasta around his penis." Another liked to eat dry oatmeal cookies before she fellated her boyfriend because he liked the prickly sensation of "crumbs and tongue." As we have seen earlier, molasses or maple syrup makes for a highly sensual medium for masturbation and oral sex (although be careful if you're counting the calories!). There are also several edible massage lotions which you can buy mail-order from marital-aid companies, such as Tasty Lovin', "the hot lickable love lotion. . . . Turn your dick into a lickable sugar-stick or your whole body into a mouthwatering dessert with this new sexy lubricant that adds a zesty flavor to your lovemaking. . . . But that's not all; it actually heats up when you blow on it . . . hot strawberry flavor!"

If you're giving oral sex to a man whose sexual history you're not quite sure of, then it's always wiser to make sure that he wears a condom to protect yourself from AIDS and other sexually transmitted diseases. But that doesn't mean you have to put up with the taste of rubber. Condoms are produced these days in an endless variety of flavors, from chocolate sundae to pina colada. I have even seen a sperm-flavored condom for women who like the taste of semen but obviously don't wish to swallow it.

Where and *when* you give your partner oral sex is just as important as *how*. An act of fellatio that may be unmemorable in bed can be transformed by choosing an unexpected moment. In a field, during a summer picnic. In a boat, in the middle of a lake. In an elevator. Lorraine, a 33-year-old driving instructor from Boston, Massachusetts, visited her husband in the hospital after he had broken both wrists in a skiing accident and gave him "the cock-sucking of a lifetime . . . long and slow, just the way I like it . . . and there was nothing he could do to stop me because both of his arms were in traction." Trudi, 28, a homemaker from Memphis, Tennessee, was tired of her boyfriend spending so long in his garage tinkering with his classic Corvette. One morning she found him lying underneath the car on an inspection trolley, with only his lower half visible. She knelt against the trolley so that he was unable to roll it out from under the car. Then she opened up his jeans and gave him oral sex. She didn't take him as far as a climax, however. She left him when he was almost there, and went back into the house. He followed her immediately, and made love to her on the family room floor. "I wanted to show him that taking care of me was much more important than taking care of that car. I needed regular lubricating, too. My breasts and my thighs were all covered with black greasy handprints, but I didn't care."

You can add all kinds of original touches to your oral sex. Janice, 27, a dressmaker from Pittsburgh, Pennsylvania, said, "One afternoon I was sitting in the bedroom sewing when my partner, Oliver, came in from the bathroom. He'd been taking a shower and he was only wearing a towel. He came over and asked me what I was doing. I said, 'Hemming, but I know what I'd *like* to be doing.' I pulled down his towel and took hold of his dick, and put it in my mouth. I've never seen him so surprised, but he was *pleasantly* surprised. His dick rose up almost at once and completely filled my mouth. I drummed against it with the tip of my tongue—I know he likes that—and at the same time I fondled his balls. He was loving it, but he said he was late, he really had to go or else his boss would give him a hard time. I said, 'You can have a much better hard time with me, and in any case, you're my prisoner.' He tried to take himself out of my mouth but I dug my fingernails into his balls and wouldn't let him go. Not that he really wanted to go.

"I kept on sucking his dick, but at the same time I picked up my sewing thread and I wound it tight around the base of his dick. Then I wound it around each of his balls, and criss-crossed it all the way up his shaft so that his flesh stood out in diamond-shaped bulges. I wound some more around the groove behind the head of his dick, and then I tied it so that it cut right into his hole. His whole dick was tied up like a parcel, just tight enough to hurt him a little, but not so tight that it was going to turn him off. I took his dick back in my mouth and sucked it and he was groaning because the bigger his dick swelled up, the tighter the thread cut into him.

"I strummed the thread that cut into his hole with the tip of my tongue—you know, like strumming a guitar string—and at the same time I pulled tight on the threads around his balls. That was too much for him. He climaxed right onto the tip of my tongue—again and again—and he shot out so much cum that it was dripping down my chin. His dick had red criss-cross marks on it afterward, but they didn't last long. But he says that he'll never forget that afternoon, not ever, even though he's not too sure he wants me to try it again."

Binding the penis with thread is a do-it-yourself version of the various devices that are used to restrict the penis during sado-masochistic sex play. The simplest of these is a leather strap that buckles tightly around the base of the penis and sometimes lifts and separates the testicles. The most complex is "six gates of hell," which is a series of leather straps or metal rings that encircle the whole length of the penis. If you're tempted to try some penis-binding of your own, make sure that the twine is not so tight that it actually breaks the skin, and never leave the binding in place for more than a few minutes.

Many men are sexually excited by pain, or at least

a limited level of pain. Love bites and back scratches increase the flow of adrenaline, and can make men feel stronger and more sexually energetic. If you find that your love life has become rather mundane, try casting yourself in the role of predatory jungle goddess. Jump on your man and tell him that you love him so much you're going to eat him, and start biting him. Not too hard—there's a very fine line between a bite that arouses and a bite that annoys—but enough to get him aroused. Be playful. Be flirtatious. But occasionally give him a nip that really makes him yelp.

Try opening his shirt and kissing and licking his nipples. Men have very sensitive nipples, and it's about time that women realized it. You can bite his nipples, too: but again, don't be unreasonable. A really hard bite on the nipples will hurt him just as much as if somebody did it to you, and believe me, he won't like it. Some men find it arousing to have clips or clothespins attached to their nipples during sex, and you could even try to introduce that into your love life if you wanted to, making it into a game of "torture."

Another highly erotic place for biting is on the side of the hip. Very few men are used to women biting them and they find the experience highly unusual and arousing. You can try biting almost anyplace at all, but the favorite spots are the backs of the shoulders; the stomach, around the navel; the buttocks; the backs of the thighs; and (believe it or not) the heels.

You can see how much this kind of sexual teasing can give you control over your sex life. As playful as it seems, it enables you to make love wherever and whenever you want, in the way that you want it. It may appear at the moment as if you're being expected to do all the work, but once your partner has begun to appreciate your sexual inventiveness, he will be inspired to be much more creative and much more attentive.

Some men are very resistant to women taking the initiative when it comes to sex. Scarlett, 28, an airline attendant from Silver Spring, Maryland, said, "Mark is very macho . . . he's a man's man. He's very virile but he doesn't have much imagination in bed. I tried a couple of things to pep up our sex life. Like once I walked into his den wearing a black lace crotchless cat suit and sat on his lap, and another time I bought a vibrator shaped like a real cock except that it was about twice the size. But both times he was angry—well, *annoyed* more than angry—as if I'd criticized his virility. When I wore the cat suit he said, 'No woman of mine has to dress like a whore to turn me on,' and when I showed him the vibrator, that was even worse. He kept on shouting, 'There's something wrong with my dick you need something like this? I'm too small, am I? Not hard enough, am I? Don't last long enough to satisfy you?' So the cat suit and the vibrator went into the trash and I've never tried anything like that again. I guess I should be grateful for having a man who loves me, but sometimes I think I'd like to try a few variations, you know, like sex in the open air, or sex in the bath, or any kind of sex apart from lying on my back staring at the ceiling."

The problem with men like Mark is that—in spite of their apparent virility—they lack confidence in their sexual aptitude. They have usually had a very conventional upbringing and often come from families in which traditional religion is very important. Their knowledge of sex and sexual technique tends to be limited to locker-room hearsay and what they've read in men's magazines, and they're frightened of trying something exotic and possibly making a fool of themselves. They have set views on what they consider to be right and wrong, and they're the kind of men who don't take kindly to criticism or ribbing. Really great sex frequently depends on having the ability to laugh at yourself—or at the very least not to lose your temper when things don't work out exactly as planned. Katrina, a 25-year-old credit controller from Orlando, Florida, said that her husband, Len, at last coaxed her into trying anal intercourse. "He had tried before but I hadn't wanted to do it. But I read this magazine article about it and it didn't seem so bad after all, so I said that he could do it if he really wanted to. He was very excited about it and when we went to bed his cock was hard already. He was very good: He didn't rush it or anything. He kissed me and caressed my breasts and he was just as tender as he always is. Then he opened up this jar of scented lubricant that he'd bought, and smeared it between the cheeks of my ass, and *that* was a very sexy feeling, I can tell you. I crouched on the bed with my butt in the air, and he slipped his finger into my asshole first. He said, 'I'm going to be real gentle with you. If it hurts at all, you just tell me.' I felt his cock up against my asshole, and I felt him pushing, but do you know what? He lost his erection. He lost it, and no matter how much he jiggled it and rubbed it he couldn't get it up again—not hard enough to push it into my asshole, anyhow. Such a buildup and then *flop*! And do you know what I like about Mark? He laughed about it. He thought it was the funniest thing.

"We actually did it later on that night, in the middle of the night, when it was dark. We were both calm and quiet. When his cock pushed into my asshole, I welcomed it, I wanted to draw it in. It went deep inside me and I felt as if my whole body was opening out, like I was space and Mark was a space traveler exploring me."

The success of Mark and Katrina's lovemaking depended not only on Katrina's willingness to try something new, but on Mark's lack of sexual pomposity. He was so tense about the idea of having anal sex with Katrina that he temporarily lost the ability to do it—and that can happen in any sexual situation. With good humor from the man and understanding from the woman, such problems can be overcome with relative ease.

If your man is more touchy than Mark about his sexual prowess, and about you taking control of your love life, don't be discouraged and don't give up trying. Make your advances much more subtle—"absentmindedly" reaching inside his open-necked shirt, for instance, when he's reading or watching TV, and then unfastening a couple of buttons so that you can touch his nipples. If you're in bed, reach over and touch his penis, but don't rush it. Play with it idly rather than trying to rub it forcibly into erection. If it begins to rise, restrain yourself. Run your fingers lightly down it and then take your hand away. When he makes love to you now, he'll feel that *he* initiated sex, rather than you. You, after all, lost interest, didn't you, and stopped stroking him? But he managed to arouse you, make love to you, and satisfy you.

Sex manuals used to make a big fuss about "erogenous zones," which are nothing more complicated than places on the body where you or your partner likes to be kissed, stroked, or caressed. Everybody has different erogenous zones of differing degrees of sensitivity. Some people, for instance, find it almost painful to have the soles of their feet tickled, while others adore it. Some men like to have their nipples pinched, others can't stand it. You can only find out your partner's favorite erogenous zones by trial and error, but there is never any harm in asking him, "Do you like that?" as you stroke the sensitive nerve endings around his hips. Equally, you should make sure that your partner knows which caresses turn you on the most, and you should never be afraid to tell him if you find some caresses ineffective or irritating. "He used to fumble with my breasts as if he was trying to solve a Rubik's cube. I just didn't know how to tell him without hurting his feelings."

Don't be afraid to experiment with erogenous zones. It's surprising what you can teach yourself about making love by trying out different techniques on your lover's body. A surprising number of men love having their closed eyes licked. And too many women ignore their partner's back. The nerve endings around the shoulder blades and down the spine are particularly sensitive, and some light caresses with fingers and/or fingernails can give him a very dreamy and pampered sense of arousal. If you slide your fingers down his back, you can reach the cleft of his buttocks, and then you can try to be even more sexually adventurous.

After his penis, your man's single most sensitive erogenous zone is his anus. Years ago, anal stimulation for men was very rarely discussed in sex manuals because of its homosexual connotations and because "real men" wouldn't openly admit that they enjoyed having things stuck up their anuses. But anal stimulation is highly pleasurable, and any woman can give her partner really great sex by learning how to excite him anally.

The simplest stimulation, of course, is stroking or tickling the anal orifice. But with practice you can learn to massage your partner's anus and give him the most extraordinary sensations. If you place the balls of your thumbs side by side on his anus and then deeply and rhythmically stroke out and away from his orifice, you will give him a feeling that he has never dreamed of. Another technique is to insert the very tip of your index finger into his anus and then roll the edge of his sphincter against the ball of your thumb, around and around. Always make sure that your fingernails are short and that you use a lubricant, even if it's only saliva.

Licking your partner's anus is another way of giving him very strong erotic feelings. This technique is traditionally known as "around the world." You can also probe into his orifice with the tip of your tongue. If your partner has showered or bathed, there is no risk that there will be any fecal matter around. The rectum is usually empty right up until the moment of defecation.

You can penetrate your partner's anus with a well-lubricated finger (or two, or even more!). You can simply slide it in and out to stimulate him, or you can reach inside to find his prostate gland, and give him a massage that will change his life forever! The best way to do this is for him to lie on his back with his legs raised and his knees apart. Insert your finger into his anus and crook it toward you (as if you were beckoning) until you can feel the soft lump of his prostate gland. Stroke it strong and slow. At the same time you can suck and fondle his penis and his testicles—although the stimulation of his prostate really makes any other caressing redundant. Men can experience a climax through prostate massage without even having an erection—a long, copious flow of semen accompanied by an overwhelming sense of well-being.

When I first started working as a sex advisor, very few men would openly admit that they masturbated. "I only buy *Playboy* for the articles." Even fewer men would admit that they stimulated themselves anally during masturbation, but of course the reality was that emergency rooms were regularly dealing with men who had inserted objects into their anuses and then discovered that they were impossible to retrieve. The German magazine *Stern* published an X-ray photograph showing a full bottle of sparkling wine inserted into a man's rectum, and the German edition of *Medical Tribune* reported on a collection of objects that surgeons at Hamburg University Clinic had removed from men's intestines over a period of five years: three massage rods, three sprayers, two vulcanite rods, a cola bottle, a boccie ball, a vacuum cleaner fitting, a chair leg, a spade handle, a candle, a radio valve, and a rolled-up copy of *Welt am Sonntag*.

As a matter of common sense, never insert anything into your partner's anus (or your own, for that matter) that carries any risk of being lost for good. In particular, never insert anything made of glass, such as a light bulb or a fluorescent tube. These days—now that our embarrassment about masturbation and anal stimulation is a thing of the past—there are all kinds of devices on the market for giving you and your partner safe anal thrills.

The simplest are the Thai love-beads—a string of small plastic beads that you can insert into your partner's anus one by one while you are making love. As he ejaculates, you pull them all out, intensifying his climax. Then there's the Anal Explorer, described on the package as "a finger-sized, whisper-smooth anal probe which penetrates with supreme ease . . . made of a translucent silicone material that quickly warms to body temperature and formed with a flattened base with finger holes for easy removal." Even more sophisticated is the Backdoor Buddy, "a flexible, super-slim, pink, penis-shaped jelly vibe that's perfect for the anal beginner . . . 7" in length, 1" in width, with a multi-speed twist control in the base for both quiet purring vibrations or shuddering deep throbs." There's even a Recto-Buzzer, which is made to a curved design in order to massage a man's prostate gland in the way we've just been discussing. Last but not least, there's the Butt Buddy, "the 7" flexi-dong . . . a remarkable new weapon for all anal lovers . . . a sleek, jelly, tapered dong with an adjustable spine that actually bends and holds to the shape you require, peach-colored and sumptuously soft."

Vibrators are also available in black, such as the Black Mamba multispeed vibrator. "If you'd like to see her eyes widen and her breath quicken, introduce her to this seven-inch ebony beast."

According to sex store proprietors and mail-order companies, more and more strap-on dildoes are being bought by women with the express purpose of doing to their lovers what their lovers have been doing to them—penetrating their anuses. Some of the dildoes are remarkably lifelike, and they give your partner the opportunity to enjoy submissive anal sex without having to resort to the services of another man. They also give *you* a further degree of control over your sex life. It's up to you to decide if and when to give your partner an anal treat; and for how long. It's up to you to decide if you're going to allow him to go all the way to a climax, or if you're going to withdraw your dildo halfway through and have him make love to you.

Mandy, a 32-year-old bank teller from Seattle, Washington, first discovered that her live-in lover, Alan, enjoyed anal sex when they took a vibrator to bed with them for *him* to use on *her*. "Alan liked to push the vibrator up my ass while he was making love to me, but that night he didn't. He just started to make love to me in the usual way—Alan on top, me underneath. We were right in the throes when my hand touched the vibrator lying next to me. Alan was really thrusting into me. I picked up the vibrator and pressed it between the cheeks of his ass, right up against his asshole, and to my surprise he didn't clench up tight, he opened up, like he really wanted it. I tried to push it in farther but he was too dry. I put the vibrator down between my legs and covered it with juice. Then I tried pushing it up his asshole again, and this time he took it right in.

"I switched the vibrator on and I could feel his cock growing even harder, right inside me. I stirred the vibrator around and he was saying things like 'oh, baby . . . oh, no . . .' and then he climaxed like somebody had given him an electric shock.

"Afterward I said, 'I didn't know ordinary men liked things up their ass.' And he said, 'Of course they do. Everybody likes it. It's just that they don't want to admit it.' So after that, I used to take out that vibrator now and then, you know, and give him a good hard poking where he liked it the most.

"Then I saw this strap-on dildo advertised. It said in the advertisement that it was made for lesbian lovers, but I know a lesbian couple and I know for sure that neither of them would use it. So anyhow, I thought, why don't I buy one and use it on Alan? He'd love it.

"When it arrived I opened it up and it looked enormous—far too big to push into Alan's asshole. It was flesh-colored, just like a real cock, with balls and everything, except that it had a kind of harness to strap it on with. I thought I'd made a terrible mistake. Like, how was I going to introduce this thing into our love life? Walk into the bedroom wearing this huge plastic cock and say, 'What do you think, darling?'

"I kept it hidden in my nightstand for over a week. But then one night we went to a wedding anniversary party and had quite a few drinks, and when we came back we were more than a little bit drunk but we were in a very amorous mood, you know? We took off our clothes and left them all over the bedroom floor. Alan got on top of me and fucked me and his cock was hard like a rock. It was great. I could twist and wriggle my hips around and yet this big hard cock was stuck right up me and I couldn't get away from it. He gave me an orgasm that night, just by fucking me, and I didn't usually find that very easy.

"He kept on fucking me even after I'd had my orgasm, and I suddenly realized that it was taking him a long time to climax because he'd had so much to drink. I said, 'Come on, it's my turn. Now I'm going to fuck *you*.' He rolled off me and I took the dildo out of the nightstand and strapped it on. He said, 'What the hell is that?' but all I said was 'you're just about to find out.' He was lying face down on the bed. I opened up a new tube of KY and I squeezed it between the cheeks of his ass, and rubbed it around, and I rubbed some on the end of the dildo, too.

"I pried the cheeks of his ass wide apart with both hands. Then I positioned the head of the dildo right up against his asshole. It was such a small hole I was sure that I'd never manage to push the dildo into it. But I pushed, and his asshole stretched, and the next thing I knew he'd taken the whole head of it into his ass. I pushed again and this time he said, 'ahh,' like it hurt him, and he reached his hand around to stop me from pushing too hard. I took the dildo out a ways, and then I pushed it again, and this time it went almost halfway in. His asshole was bright red and it was stretched so wide I almost felt sorry for him. But he was loving it . . . he was loving the pain, and he was loving the fact that I was fucking him. I fondled his balls and then I started to jerk his cock. He was so turned on that juice was actually dripping out of the end of his cock, and I rubbed it all down his cock and around his balls. I leaned forward and pushed the dildo in farther, and then farther still, and then it was right inside him, right up his ass, as far as it would go, all nine inches of it.

"I fucked him very slow, partly because I didn't want to hurt him, and partly because I wanted him to have as much pleasure as possible before he came to a climax. The dildo made a sticky, sucking sound in his ass. Once or twice I took it right out and his asshole was gaping wide, and kind of wincing like it was begging to have it back. I swung my breasts against his back so that he could feel my nipples. I fucked him for nearly ten minutes, and slowly massaged his cock, and I think he was amazing for holding out so long. But in the end he started to climax and there was nothing that anybody could have done to stop him. His ass gripped the dildo like a vise. His balls went tight. And suddenly he was pumping sperm all over the bed and he kept on saying, 'Oh my God, oh my God, oh . . .' like he couldn't believe it was happening."

What did Mandy think about her lover's liking anal penetration? "I think it's normal. If he did it with another man maybe I wouldn't think it was quite so normal. But if anal sex makes women feel good, why shouldn't a man feel the same way? And more than that, you can't even describe the power of it, the sheer power of gripping a man from behind and fucking his ass, and knowing that *you're* in charge, *you're* making all the moves, and that he's taking it from you because you're turning him on so much."

Did it lead her to respect him any less? "No, the opposite. I admire people who can give themselves. I admire men who can open up to me, whether they do it emotionally or whether they can do it physically, or both."

Too many sexual relationships gradually fall apart because couples keep their distance from each other, and won't allow their partner to be privy to their private fantasies. They never tell each other what they really want, and this is especially true of men. A woman can bridge that distance by giving her lover constant coaxing, constant flirtation, and encouraging him to think about lovemaking at times when he normally wouldn't even be *dreaming* about lovemaking. Those so-called "surveys" which suggest that men think about sex every three minutes of the day are completely without scientific foundation. As one young wife told me, "If he thinks about it so much, why doesn't he do it? I'm here, I'm ready, I'm always willing. If he thinks about anything every three minutes of the day, it's the World Series."

So let's turn now to ways in which you can ignite your partner's sexual interest and keep it alight—so that he can warm you just when you need him the most.

Secret 6: Play Sexy for Me

Sex is serious: It's the strongest expression of love that two people can show for each other. But just because it's serious in that respect, it doesn't mean that you or your partner have to take it too seriously. As we saw in the last chapter, joy and laughter are important ingredients in any relationship, and that includes a sexual relationship.

Sex can be passionate, intense, dramatic. Sex can be the path to intellectual enlightenment. But sex is also play. It's a recreation. And one of the secrets of really great sex is for you and your partner to develop a sense of mischief when you make love, a sense of fun.

Delia, 24, a cosmetician from Detroit, Michigan, had a two-year relationship with a married man called Scott and became pregnant. The relationship ended when her son was born. Now she is living on her own but has a new lover, Vincent. "My affair with Scott was always very serious, yes. He wasn't at all happy at home and I guess he used me to try to bring some excitement into his life. Not that our relationship was ever exciting. We met in hotel rooms and had sex, and then we went down to the bar and Scott drank too much and told me how miserable his life was, and how he wished he could get a divorce and marry me. I liked him. I loved him, if I'm going to admit the truth, and I think in a very selfish way he loved me, too. But our relationship was nothing but stress and problems. He was using his affair with me to punish his wife and he was using her pain to punish himself, and I knew in my heart that he was never going to leave her. The day I told him that I was pregnant, I thought—I hoped—that he might leave her then. But there was always some problem that stopped him from going. One of the kids had to go to the orthodontist. The dog needed grooming. His wife had come down with the flu, and as much as he hated her he had to stay at home and nurse her.

"In the end, I had to break it off. It hurt me so bad, but I had to. I broke it off and I didn't answer any of his calls. And it was only about a week later that I went bowling with my friend Naomi and I met Vincent. Vincent is just the opposite of Scott. He's single, he's funny. He's never been worried about going back home on time. He doesn't lie to me, either, the way Scott did. I think an affair can survive a whole lot of ups and downs so long as people don't lie to each other. Vincent doesn't seem to mind my baby, either. He doesn't try to be a father to him, but he's very affectionate, you know, and he rocks him to sleep if I'm busy with cooking or something.

"Vincent and I first made love about a week after we met. He came around to my apartment and I cooked him a pasta carbonara. We lay on the floor by the fire with a bottle of wine and listened to some blues and then we got to kissing. The next thing I knew we were naked and we were making love. When we met, Vincent wasn't at all experienced, not like Scott. He'd had lots of girlfriends but of course they'd all been very young. He's beautiful looking: thin, with an angelic face. He has this crucifix of silky black hair on his chest, and silky black pubic hair, and a long, long cock with a foreskin, which I'd never seen on a man before, and I thought it was *fascinating*. I could have played with it all night, rolling it back and rolling it forward.

"He was sexy, but he didn't have any idea how to please a woman properly. He used to kiss me and hold me, but then he always got too impatient and wanted to start fucking before I was ready. I'm one of these women who takes a long time to get aroused. When I am, I think I'm dynamite, but it takes me a long, long time; and most nights, Vincent was finished and fast asleep before I was even half warmed up.

"It got so that I was frustrated most of the time, and we started to argue. But I thought to myself, What can I tell him? How do you tell a man that you adore him, and that he's sexy, and that you don't want to break up with him, but at the same time tell him that he's not much good in bed?"

I suggested to Delia that she try to get Vincent out of the usual bedroom scenario and develop some sex games with him. He was still young enough to have a strong sense of play, and so it wouldn't be too difficult for her to improve his lovemaking skills without him being aware that he was being "taught." The first game I suggested was "tease-and-chase," in which your partner really has to work at catching you and making love to you. You *can* play this game in your bedroom, or around the house, but it is much more effective if you can find a location outdoors, with unlimited space.

Delia was lucky in having several hundred acres of woodland close to her home. "I made a picnic—nothing special, just some cold chicken and salad and a couple of bottles of wine—and we drove out into the woods. It was a beautiful warm summer's afternoon, perfect. We spread two blankets on the ground next to a small lake. We sat on the blankets and talked for a while but Vincent was in a very horny mood and he kept kissing me and touching my breasts, and after a while he said, 'Come on, let's make love.' I said, 'No, I'm going to take a swim first.' And that did take some self-discipline, you know, because I was feeling very horny, too. Anyhow, I undressed, except for my panties, and waded into the lake. The water was great, it was really warm. I swam around a little and then Vincent came in after me. He was naked and his cock was sticking out like a flagpole. He came swimming up to me and kissed me, and then he started caressing me under the water, fondling my nipples and trying to get his hands into my panties. I kept feeling his stiff cock up against my stomach and I was aching to touch it, but I didn't. I gave him a kiss and then I swam back to shore.

"He came wading out of the water after me and caught me. He kissed me some more and tried to pull my panties down but I managed to struggle free. We were both laughing like crazy. Vincent kept saying, 'I want you! I want you!' He looked beautiful—completely naked, his hair all wet. I tried to run past him and up the bank but he caught me and both of us fell over into the mud at the edge of the lake. I was thrashing and kicking and both of us rolled over and over until we were plastered in mud. Vincent got on top of me and smeared mud all over my breasts and down my sides. I took a big wet handful of mud and wiped it all over his stomach. Then I smothered his cock and his balls with mud, and rubbed him up and down. It was so sexy the way the pink head of his cock kept peeping out of his brown muddy foreskin.

"He pulled down my panties, which was quite difficult because they were all wet and thick with sticky brown mud. I said, 'We're going to have to wash ourselves first.' So we got up and dived back into the lake, and swam around a little more to get ourselves clean. Vincent came up to me and held me close, and touched my cunt underwater. He stroked my clitoris and then he pushed his finger up inside me. I think he would have fucked me right there, in the middle of the lake, but I fell back in the water and splashed him, and then I waded away.

"I ran up the bank and into the woods. Vincent came after me. I tried to hide behind a tree but he came around behind me and caught me. He pinned me against the tree and held my hands up above my head and kissed me. Then he picked me up, right off the ground, and pulled my cunt wide open with his fingers, and lowered me onto his cock. It went in so deep that I felt as if it was going to come out of my mouth. He was skinny, but he was very strong, and he was able to lift me up so that his cock was almost out of my cunt, and then let me back down again. We were both beginning to be very turned on by now. Well, I know how much I was, whereas if we'd fucked on the blankets the minute he wanted to have sex, I wouldn't have been turned on at all, not very much, anyhow.

"He couldn't hold me for very long, but those minutes were amazing . . . being lifted up and down on a man's erect cock as if I didn't weigh anything at all. The sun shining, the birds singing, the breeze blowing between my legs so that I could feel how wet my cunt was. It was heaven, but of course it couldn't last forever. Vincent let me down on the ground, in a heap of dead leaves. He knelt down between my thighs with his cock in his hand and he was about to carry on fucking me when I rolled myself around and took his cock in my mouth. It was delicious. It tasted like me. I sucked on it and played with his balls and even though he wanted to keep on fucking me there wasn't any way that he was going to stop me from doing *this*.

"I slid right down between his thighs and licked his balls and his asshole and kept on rubbing his cock. I opened my legs up, too, so that he was staring right at my cunt, and it was then that he got the message. He leaned forward and started to lick my clitoris, and that was what I wanted. That was so incredibly arousing that I closed my eyes and I almost forgot that I was supposed to be licking him, too. His tongue flipped my clitoris and then he delicately poked the tip of it into my pee hole, which is the strangest feeling, and then on down to my vagina. All the time he was licking me I could feel the sun shining warm on my open cunt and that breeze blowing.

"I sucked Vincent's cock harder and I knew that an orgasm was coming. It's like hearing a train in the distance and you know that it's coming to run you down no matter what you do. Vincent kept on licking my clitoris faster and faster. I had my mouth full of cock but I wasn't sucking or licking any more, I was panting. My hips started to spasm. Then he gave me one last lick and I was jerking and jumping around on those leaves and I felt as if the world had ended.

"Vincent didn't even wait for me to stop trembling. He took his cock out of my mouth and plunged it right into my cunt, all the way up, and started to fuck me. I had another orgasm, and another. I didn't know whether I liked it or not, but I couldn't stop myself. Then Vincent slowed down . . . slower and slower. I looked up at his face and his eyes were closed and his mouth was open. I touched his lips with my fingers and stroked his cheek. He was right on the very edge of coming and he wanted to make it last longer, that was why he was fucking me so slow.

"He opened his eyes and kissed me, and then without a word he took his cock out of me and stood up. He rubbed his cock two or three times and sperm spurted out of it and dropped all over my stomach and my breasts. When he was finished he knelt down beside me and massaged the sperm into my nipples and all around my navel. A drop of sperm was still dangling from the end of his cock so I leaned forward and licked it up. I said, 'You don't know what you did to me today. It was amazing.' He didn't say anything but I could tell that he was pleased with himself. He'd discovered how to turn me on and how to give me an orgasm, even though I hadn't done anything to criticize him or make him feel clumsy and inexperienced."

If you can *show* your partner the effects of creative, exciting, and considerate lovemaking, the likelihood is that he will try to repeat the performance next time, and hopefully improve on it. Everybody needs reassurance that they're good in bed, but we don't always have the vocabulary to tell each other how much we appreciated a really satisfying fuck . . . not without sounding either mawkish or crude. At least we're not as badly off for sex words as some other countries. When I write articles about sex for Poland, for example, they have to translate "cunt" as "butterfly" or "little flower" since they have no slang word for a woman's private parts that isn't so coarse as to be publicly unmentionable. If you're partner's given you a good time, try to think of something to say that will let him know how you feel, but you can communicate your satisfaction even more eloquently by continuing to hold him close, by caressing him, and continuing to fondle his penis, even though it's soft. Too many couples spring apart as soon as their lovemaking is over, and go on doing what they were doing before as if nothing had happened. I know that you can often feel too hot and sweaty for a very close embrace, but do try to continue some kind of physical contact. Run your fingers through his hair. Lick his shoulder. Play with his nipples. And don't just smile—*beam.* You're that cat that got the cream, remember.

Apart from running through the woods playing hide-and-go-seek, there are plenty of other games you can play to prolong your lovemaking. "My husband makes Speedy Gonzales look slow," complained one bride of eighteen months. "Sometimes I haven't had time to make myself halfway comfortable before he's finished." However, we're not necessarily talking about premature ejaculation here—the problem of men who can't stop themselves from climaxing too soon. There are ways in which premature ejaculation can be successfully overcome. The simplest of these is for the man to distract himself during sexual intercourse by thinking about something totally unrelated to sex. Probably the most effective is the squeeze technique devised by sex researchers Masters & Johnson. I have described it in detail in earlier books, but basically it involves the man taking his penis out of his partner's vagina when he feels that ejaculation is imminent, at which point she presses the ball of her thumb against his urethral opening and squeezes him hard until the feeling subsides.

We're talking here about men who are sexually selfish—men who don't devote any time to making sure that their partners are fully aroused before lovemaking and well satisfied afterward. I'm not saying that they're all *deliberately* selfish. Most of the time they're not even aware that they're doing anything wrong. But whether they know it or not, the effect on you is just the same. Peremptory, unsatisfactory sex can leave you feeling frustrated and unloved.

I often recommend that a woman in this situation play the massage game. All she has to do is buy herself some massage oil and teach herself some basic massage techniques. (There are dozens of very good instructional books on the subject.) If she offers to give her partner a massage before they go to bed, this will delay intercourse and introduce a new and very sensual element of love play. Once she has massaged *him,* she can ask him to try and massage *her,* encouraging him to make his manipulations increasingly sexual—shoulders, breasts, thighs, buttocks, and eventually a gentle clitoral massage.

Susanne, 29, who works for a computer company in Cincinnati, Ohio, said, "Rob really looks forward to his massage these days. He works very hard in a high-stress job and he comes home at night with his muscles all knotted up. Before, he used to get into bed, climb on top of me and that was that. It was the tension of his job, mostly. He made love to me like that because he needed to get rid of the stress and get rid of it quick. Now he's much more relaxed and laid-back, and he enjoys giving me a massage, too, especially when it gets to the intimate bits! It's so sensual being covered in sweet-smelling oil . . . you can slide your hands all over your partner's body, and you can slip in your fingers wherever you like without having to worry about saliva or extra lubricant."

Another way to slow down your partner's sexual haste is to acquire a vibrator and ask him to use it on you. If you think that his reaction might be hostile, or if you're too embarrassed to admit that you bought it yourself, you can always tell him a little white lie and say that your friends gave it to you as a practical joke— "because I'm always saying how much I miss your lovemaking when you're away." Again, there's nothing like lightheartedness to disarm any sexual tension.

Vibrators come in so many exotic shapes and sizes and varieties these days that it's difficult to make a recommendation. But judging from the opinions of all the women with whom I had sexual discussions while preparing this book, three particular vibrators seem more arousing than most. The most popular is Mr. Softee, a bright pink penis made of soft jelly vinyl—"feels firm yet ideally supple"—which is supplied with or without a vibrating electric motor. Second is a replica penis based on the legendary sexual organs of black video star Sean Michael. "Sculpted from his actual penis, this black masterpiece is guaranteed to make her gulp! Over 10 inches in length and detailed with every vein and wrinkle." Third is a newcomer, a vibrator made to look like an enormous cucumber. "Seven inches of green knobby delights, with a mushy firmness that will send a quiver through her body as you drive it home!"

With a vibrator to play with, your partner will be much less inclined to hurry straight into intercourse, and you will benefit from all the pleasure it can give you. Jodi, a 33-year-old cab driver from Schaumburg, Illinois, explained that her husband, Kieran, had become less and less bothered about love play, and that he often made love to her in the middle of the night when she was asleep. "I wake up to find his cock inside me, and him pounding away like a jackhammer. He comes, and rolls over, and the next thing I know he's asleep, and I've only just woken up. I'm raring for it, and he's unconscious." Part of the problem was caused by the fact that Kieran had a physically demanding job during the day loading cargo at the airport, and when he first came home he was always exhausted. His sexual urges didn't awaken until he had slept for four or five hours, by which time Jodi was deeply asleep. "I knew he loved me, and he didn't mean to leave me feeling so frustrated, but our relationship wasn't working at all, and I had to do something about it."

Jodi bought a penis-shaped vibrator. "I showed it to Kieran and he said, 'What's this? I'm not satisfying you or something?' But I said, 'Listen, *you* like having sex in the middle of the night and I like having it before I go to sleep.' He said, 'I'm too tired to have sex at that time of the evening. I don't even think I could get it up.' So I said, 'That's why I bought the vibrator. You can spend five or ten minutes giving me some satisfaction before I go to sleep, and then I won't feel so bad when you make love to me in the middle of the night."

Jodie wasn't sure how Kieran was going to react, but my experience is that if you offer a man a previously thought-out solution to a sex problem, he'll usually accept it without too much hesitation. The only word of caution I'll give about vibrators is that you must make it clear to your partner that *he's* the focus of your sexual excitement, not this disembodied vinyl penis. You don't want him to feel that he can't quite satisfy you, unlike this ever-rigid creation with its battery-operated buzzer. For that reason, give the vibrator to him, and let him use it on you. Don't give him one-woman one-vibrator demonstrations of sexual self-stimulation in which he's nothing but an uninvolved spectator. You may be able to do this later when your problems are sorted out and your partner feels more secure about your vibrator, but to begin with it's important to make him feel that the vibrator is *his*—something that he can use to give you greater sexual stimulation.

"We went to bed and Kieran left the vibrator on the table next to the alarm clock. I didn't know whether he was going to try it at first. But then he picked it up and turned it this way and that and said, 'Do you think I ought to be jealous of it?' I laughed and said, 'Never . . . it doesn't have a word of conversation.' He switched it on and it hummed. 'Feels strange,' he said. But I said, 'I always had a fantasy about you having two cocks. Now you do.'

I tugged open the ribbons in the front of my nightdress so that my breasts were bare. I said, 'Why don't you try it on my breasts? It's supposed to make them firmer.' He touched the vibrator's head against my nipples. He was right; the vibration was real strange, but it was exciting, too. It buzzed through my nipples and made them stiffen up, and when Kieran rolled the whole vibrator around my breasts it gave me this feeling that they were tingling. 'Do you like that?' he asked me, and he kissed me. I said, 'It's weird. I never felt anything like it before, but I think it's turning me on.' I lifted my nightdress and put my hand down between my legs and I was so wet that I couldn't believe it. I rubbed my fingers into my pussy and then I brought them up and showed them to Kieran. 'Look what you've done to me already.' Then I rubbed my pussy juice all around my nipples, and Kieran pressed the vibrator up against them, and flipped them from side to side. He had never spent so much time fondling my breasts for years, and my nipples began to feel as if they were buzzing, too, like having two bees instead of nipples.

"Kieran moved the vibrator downward. My thighs were close together but he slipped it in between them. He let it creep slowly upward, still vibrating, and the insides of my thighs began to tingle in the same way that my breasts had, and I had a feeling in my clitoris that I just can't describe to you.

"He brought it right up against my pussy and held it there. It was warm now, and it felt almost like a real cock, except that it was buzzing! Kieran ran it up and down my pussy slit so that it was covered in juice. Then he opened up my legs and placed the head of the vibrator right between my lips. He said, 'How would you like me to fuck you, ma'am? Fast or slow?' and he pushed that vibrator up inside my pussy so slow that inside of my head I was begging him to push it up faster. I wanted more. I wanted more. I wanted it up right up inside me, buzzing inside my pussy! It had such a big fat cock head on it, it was bigger than a real cock, and I could feel every bump on it. I kept squeezing my pussy muscles around it and the feeling was just sensational.

"I shut my eyes. I was sweating and I was panting and I was digging my nails into Kieran's shoulders. My pussy was so wet that the sheet between my legs was soaked. The juice was flooding out of me so that I felt as if I was wetting myself, even though I wasn't. Kieran kept on sliding that vibrator in and out of me, and at the same time he was flicking my clitoris with his finger. He was touching me so lightly that I could hardly feel him, and that was so *tantalizing,* you know? He was giving me this feeling that an orgasm was there, an orgasm was nearly there, but I couldn't quite reach it.

"It was then that he took the vibrator out of me and knelt between my legs. I opened my eyes and looked down and his cock was rearing up. He opened my legs even wider and he slid his cock into my pussy, all the way in, right up to his big hairy balls, and that was all it took to make me come. It was wonderful. The best orgasm ever known. His cock didn't vibrate inside me but it was big and hard and it was his, and I held him tight and I knew that things were going to get better."

Kieran and Jodie still experience some problems with their sexual relationship. Sometimes Kieran is genuinely too tired to make love early in the evening. When that happens, Jodie amuses herself by lying next to him, fondling his penis, while she uses the vibrator to stimulate herself. "I don't hide it. I lie there with my legs wide open pushing the vibrator in and out of my pussy, and Kieran knows that I'm doing it. Sometimes he stirs himself and makes love to me. Sometimes he just touches me and strokes my hair while I'm masturbating. Sometimes he's totally bushed and he doesn't even open his eyes. He still makes love to me in the middle of the night, but when he does, he always gives me the chance to wake up, kissing my breasts or licking my pussy . . . lots of foreplay, very gentle . . . and sometimes he uses the vibrator. Two nights ago he woke me at three-thirty in the morning. He had his cock in my pussy, and the vibrator right up my ass. And do you know what woke me? He switched the vibrator on, and I had this buzzing feeling deep inside me, and I didn't know what it was. I think it was probably the feeling of two people making the best of a difficult situation, because they love each other."

The relief that people feel when they manage to

put aside their sexual inhibitions is extraordinary. When a couple realize that they can tell each other anything, and do anything at all in front of each other, the sense of release can rekindle not only their sex life but all of their feelings of love and attachment. There was no doubt that Kieran was surprised when Jodie presented him with a vibrator, if not shocked, but after he had understood what it could do to improve their sexual relationship, he welcomed it into his bed. Jodie wasn't altogether satisfied, and there continued to be times when she felt like sex and he couldn't give it to her. But at least she was masturbating instead of having an affair with another man. Whatever your partner's reaction to the appearance in your bedroom of a replica penis, you can assure him that a replica is very much less threatening than the real thing.

Another game that can help you to take control of your sex life, believe it or not, is bondage. You might be asking how it's possible to take control of anything at all when you're handcuffed, or lying on a bed with your wrists and ankles tied and a blindfold over your eyes, and maybe a gag in your mouth, too. But your sheer helplessness demands that your partner do something sexually inventive to stimulate you. It puts him completely in charge of your sexual pleasure, without your help. It confronts him with the challenge of arousing you in ways that he may not normally have been inspired to try if you were simply lying in bed next to him.

When you agree to take part in bondage, you are tacitly saying to your partner, "I agree to let you explore me and arouse me in any way you want." Of course this doesn't include inflicting any kind of pain or injury, and if you do want him to keep within certain limits you should make that clear before you start—such as no anal penetration or no wet sex.

There are strict codes to which anyone who decides to try bondage should religiously adhere. The most important of these is that you should have a prearranged signal for instant release. No questions asked, the second you give or get that signal, the game is instantly over. You should never do anything to restrict your own breathing or your partner's breathing. Both men and women can intensify their sexual climax by half-choking themselves, but the risks far outweigh the benefits, and every year there are literally hundreds of fatalities caused by pleasure-seekers who went too far. Somebody in bondage should never be left alone, not even for a few seconds, and you should never practice bondage by yourself.

Given these precautions, bondage can be an entertaining and highly erotic game that allows you to go beyond the normal inhibitions of an everyday sexual relationship. It can give you that feeling of being sexually dominated by your partner while at the same time obliging him to be more attentive to your needs.

Pammie, a 26-year-old personal assistant from Scottsdale, Arizona, said that while her partner, Tim, made love to her regularly, "he always seems to be making love for his own enjoyment, you know, rather than mine." Specifically she complained that although he enjoyed plenty of loveplay and didn't rush into intercourse, he didn't concentrate on the kind of erotic stimulation that would have aroused *her*. "Everything he does to me, he does to turn *himself* on, rather than me. I have very big breasts, and I love having them touched and fondled, especially my nipples, which are very, very sensitive. Tim loves my breasts, he's always saying what a turn-on they are, but his favorite way of fondling my breasts is to press them tightly together and push his cock into my cleavage. He says it's almost as good as fucking my cunt, but it doesn't do very much for me. Then again he likes to hold his cock up against my lips so that I can lick it, and when it's wet he can slide it from side to side like he's putting lipstick on me. He loves it when I kiss his balls and scratch his butt with my fingernails, but he never does anything like that to me. He hardly ever touches my cunt before we make love and he never goes down on me and licks it.

"By the time he puts himself inside me, he's so turned on that he's almost ready to come, but I'm always way behind him. I love it when he makes loves to me, but it never lasts long enough, and by the time he climaxes I'm not even halfway there. I usually end up quietly masturbating in the middle of the night, just to satisfy myself."

The key to Pammie's problem was to turn Tim's attention away from his own pleasure and direct it to hers. There were several possible ways of doing this. One was for Pammie to play harder to get, and physically to wriggle out of situations such as Tim inserting his penis into her cleavage, or rubbing it up against her lips. She was being far too submissive by allowing him to do this without giving her the stimulation she wanted in return. If she wanted him to give her oral sex, she could have opened her legs and parted her vaginal lips and invited him to taste her. Not very subtle, perhaps, but he could hardly have missed the point. Incidentally, if you like oral sex and feel that your partner isn't giving you enough of it, then it's worth trimming or shaving off your pubic hair. Almost every man I spoke to during the preparation of this book said that he not only preferred giving oral sex (cunnilingus) to a woman with a hairless vulva, but that its visual appeal alone was a strong incentive to do it. "You can kiss it like a mouth, and you can suck the lips without choking on hair."

Another way for Pammie to redirect Tim's sexual attention would have been for her to take hold of his hands during loveplay and physically guide them onto her nipples and between her legs. She could have accompanied this with a little play-acting, murmuring with pleasure as he fondled her, and telling him how much she liked it when he touched her there. However, this technique doesn't always meet with the man's wholehearted approval. Some men resent being told or shown what to do, especially when it comes to sex. And it was important for Tim to create his own ways of turning Pammie on, so that he felt proud of himself. That was the only way in which he was going to improve his lovemaking technique, and improve it permanently.

So one evening Pammie suggested they try bondage. But Tim said, 'You're not tying me to any bed.' But I said, 'No, I didn't mean you. I meant me. I could be your helpless prisoner, couldn't I, and you could do whatever you wanted to me.' Tim didn't say anything more about it, so when he came to bed I handed him some of my scarves and said, 'How about it? Tying me up, I mean.' So he said, 'Okay . . .' He undressed me except for my bra and my little see-through panties, which were black nylon, edged with black lace. He led me over to the bed. He tied my wrists to the brass rails at the head of the bed, and my ankles to the two posts at the bottom of the bed, so that my arms were outstretched and my legs were wide apart. He leaned over me and kissed me, and then he ran his finger between my legs and said, 'That's a very naughty pair of panties you're wearing. I can see your cunt through them. I think you'll have to be punished for that.' He picked up another scarf and wrapped it tightly around my eyes so that I couldn't see. Then he took another scarf and gagged me with it, so I couldn't speak, either. I'd been expecting him to do that—but I didn't expect what he did next. He took my earplugs out of my nightstand drawer and plugged up both of my ears, so that I was blind and dumb and deaf, too. It was the strangest sensation—frightening, in a way, but very sexual, too. I felt totally vulnerable, and for a moment I thought I was going to panic. But then I felt Tim kiss my cheek, and nuzzle my neck, and that was very reassuring.

"I felt something cold and metal between my breasts. At first I thought it was a knife, and I thought, he's not going to hurt me, is he? I suddenly realized I didn't know very much about him, about his family background, about who he really was. Then my bra fell apart and bared my breasts and I realized that he'd cut it with a pair of scissors. My bra! I couldn't believe it. But there was absolutely nothing I could do.

"I felt him touching my nipples and rolling them between his fingers. Then I felt his tongue making circles around them, and flicking them. He took them between his teeth and stretched them, and at the same time he licked the end of them with the tip of his tongue. He hadn't ever done anything like that to me before. I guess he felt a sense of power, you know, from having me all tied up, and he was really going to take advantage of it. Which in actual fact was fine by me, because I loved having my nipples tugged and bitten like that. It was even better when he cupped both hands around my breast and slowly massaged it.

"He spent more time playing with my breasts than he ever had before, even when we were first having sex. He squeezed them and he licked them and he rubbed his hair against them . . . that's sensational, that feeling. Then I felt something else, something hard and warm. He was massaging my breasts with his cock, and rolling my nipples against his balls. My breasts are so sensitive that once or twice I've had an orgasm just from having my nipples fondled. It doesn't happen very often but it nearly happened that day.

"Tim ran his tongue down my stomach and licked my navel. Then I felt his hand inside my panties. He didn't take them off, but I felt a kind of tugging, and then I felt his fingers on my cunt and I realized what he must have done . . . he had cut open the crotch of my panties with his scissors.

"Once he had cut a hole, he tore the nylon wide apart and exposed my cunt. He slipped his hand inside and massaged me, around and around. My cunt was incredibly juicy and I could feel him spreading the juice all around my thighs and in between the cheeks of my ass. He opened my cunt up wide, and then he started to lick it. You don't have any idea how sexy that is, when you can't see and you can't hear and you can't break free. Your lover's licking your cunt and you can't do anything about it, nothing at all. You can't tell him to hurry, you can't tell him anything. All you can do is lie back and feel that warm, wet tongue going lap, lap, lap on your clitoris and slithering its way down to your cunt hole and poking at your ass.

"While he licked me, he reached up with one hand and fondled my breasts. With the other hand, he stroked my cunt lips and dipped his finger into my cunt. I felt one finger, then two. Then one of the fingers was taken out. A moment later, I felt it touching my asshole. He must have dipped it into my cunt just to lubricate it. I didn't know whether I wanted to let it into my asshole or not, but I didn't have any choice. My asshole was too slippery with juice to stop him from pushing his finger inside, and it went all the way in, right up to the knuckle. He stirred it around and around and the feeling was weird, but what a turn-on! And all the time his tongue was lapping at my clitoris.

"I started to have mini-orgasms. I couldn't help myself. My whole body felt as if it was just about to explode. My nipples felt as if they were on fire, they were so sensitive, and I would have done anything to have my hands free so that I could stretch my cunt lips wide apart and rub Tim's face into it. But I couldn't. All I could do was jump up and down with these mini-orgasms, and bite the scarf that was gagging me. I was desperate to have a huge great orgasm; and at the same time I wanted this all to go on forever. Tim had never turned me on like this before. I was so aroused I felt like I was going mad.

"It was then that I lost control of my bladder and peed all over myself. I felt humiliated but at the same time it excited me all the more, because there was nothing I could do about it. I could feel it running everywhere. Tim stopped licking me and knelt up between my legs so that my pee splashed all over his cock and his balls. He waited until I had completely finished, and then he plunged his wet cock right into my cunt, all the way in. It was enormous, and so hard, like it was carved out of solid wood.

"He fucked me for so long that my cunt began to get sore. I don't exactly know how long it was—maybe fifteen or twenty minutes. But somehow he managed to stop himself from coming, and he gave me orgasm after orgasm until I lost count and I was praying for him to stop, but also praying for him *not* to stop. At last I felt him climaxing into my cunt, and I had *another* orgasm, even though I didn't want to. I must have had about twelve or thirteen, one after the other.

"Tim kissed me all over—my feet, my knees, my thighs, my cunt, my stomach, my breasts—and then he loosened my gag and kissed me on the lips. I think we were both too shaken to say anything. I mean, this wasn't just sex, this wasn't just two people fucking. This was like, something *spiritual*, you know? This was two people getting into each other's souls."

When you play any kind of sex game with your partner, you give yourselves permission to do things that you otherwise might never have had the nerve to try. A game is one of the best ways of breaking down your inhibitions because you're not really being *you,* you're acting a part, and if anything goes wrong, it's your game-character who's responsible. You're role-playing, which means that you can do almost anything you want without being blamed for it. I've come across couples who play all kinds of varieties of sexual games, from a naked romp on the beach to a full sub/dom session in the basement with black leather and whips and hot candlewax dropped onto bare nipples.

If you want to improve your sexual relationship with your partner, and you want to get into some really great sex, then see if you can devise a game which will sexually excite him, but at the same time make him realize that he could be much more active and creative in bed. In other words, come up with a game that will show him what he's missing. As Pammie found out, it's more than worth the effort. After that first night of bondage, Tim's sexual attitude changed completely, because he had discovered that giving other people erotic pleasure is an erotic pleasure in itself.

Now let's go on to the limits of sexual stimulation, and see how you can explore them and enjoy them without fear and without embarrassment, and how you can teach your lover to give you the absolute ultimate in really great sex.

Secret 7: Boldly Go . . . to the Final Frontier

Your meditation sessions should have helped you to relax your inhibitions about adventurous sex, but there is still no substitute for trying it and seeing how much you enjoy it. Most of the time I find that couples remain sexually conservative for the simple reason that neither of them actually comes out and says what he or she would like to try.

Marcia, a 34-year-old teacher from San Diego, California, said that she had found out only by accident that her husband, Len, had always had an urge to make love to her outside, not necessarily on a beach or in a forest; their own backyard would have excited him just as much. She had been in the shower and had forgotten that she had left her towels hanging outside to dry, so she had stepped naked into the yard to bring them in.

"I hadn't even realized that Len had seen me. I thought he was in his den, working. But while I was taking down the towels I suddenly felt his arms around me. I said, '*Len,* not now!' But I couldn't stop him. He turned me around and he kissed me, and he ran his hands all over me. My nipples were standing up stiff and that wasn't just because of the breeze, either! Len dropped the towels onto the patio and spread them out. Then he took off his shirt and his pants and before I knew it he was naked, too. His cock was sticking up and his balls were all tight and wrinkled. He said, 'Come on,' and pulled me down onto the towels. He was urgent but he wasn't rough. I said, 'We can't do it here . . . supposing the neighbors look over the fence?' But all he said was, 'Maybe they'll learn something.' He laid me down and kissed me, and then he fondled my breasts and kissed my nipples. I was a little frightened, but I was very excited, too. He kissed me all the way down my body, and then he opened up my legs and kissed my vagina. It felt fabulous in the open air . . . ten times more sensitive, and I could really feel the wetness, too.

"He pushed his cock inside me and made love to me so strongly. It was wonderful to feel the sun on his back. He was so energetic and his cock was so hard it was just like the times we used to make love when we first got together. When he came, I came, too, and I hadn't been able to do that for years.

"Afterward we just lay on our backs feeling the

sun on our naked bodies. I reached over and played with his cock and it wasn't long before it started to stiffen up again. The second time we made love, we did it real slow, and neither of us came, but it was sensational, it really was. Now we make love outdoors whenever we can. We've done it on the seashore, we've done it in the woods, we've done it in the desert. We did it on a golf course once, right on the green. We still do it in the backyard. Once we even did it when it was raining, and that was amazing. I was on top, and Len pulled the cheeks of my bottom wide apart so that I could feel the rain on my anus. I just wish that it would rain more often, but that's California for you!

"Len had been turned on by the idea of making love in the open air ever since he had seen nudist magazines when he was younger. I asked him why he had never suggested making love in the open air before. He didn't really know, except he thought that I probably wouldn't like the idea. But, as you've guessed, I love it; and it's livened up our sex life amazingly, because we're always trying to think of new places to make love. I can recommend it to anyone."

Another sexual attraction for which men are often too reserved to ask is for you to walk around naked at unexpected times and in unexpected places. As we have seen, men are highly responsive to visual stimuli, and there is nothing more visually stimulating for your partner than your naked body. Nudity around the house has an innocent eroticism about it: You haven't undressed specifically for sex, but simply because you enjoy walking around the house with no clothes on and you enjoy showing yourself off to the man you love.

Helen, a 25-year-old accountant from Pittsburgh, Pennsylvania, tried it with her partner Steve. "We bought a new car and Steve started to spend every Saturday morning washing and waxing it. Before that we always spent the whole of Saturday morning in bed reading the papers and watching television and making love. It was one of my favorite mornings of the whole week, because we both work very long hours and we didn't often get together like that.

"So one morning, when I got up to make the coffee, I didn't put on my nightdress or anything. I could see Steve looking at me but he didn't say anything. When I brought in the coffee he leaned forward and gave me a kiss, and said, 'You look beautiful, but aren't you cold?' I said, 'Not at all. In fact, I'm hot.' I climbed back into bed and he turned over and started to kiss me and caress me. I could feel his dick up against my thigh and it was hard and springy. He felt my breasts and then he turned me over and fucked me from behind. It wasn't exactly rape but he was very forceful. He held on to my hips and pulled me down with every stroke so that his dick went in deeper. I loved it: It was just like those mornings we used to have before we bought the car.

"But afterward he finished his coffee and said, 'That's it . . . I gotta give baby her weekly bath,' and he got out of bed and pulled on his jeans and his T-shirt and went down to wash the car. I wasn't going to let him get away so easy. I followed him out of the house completely naked, and he was already out there with a bucket of Turtle Wax, sudsing the roof. He said, 'Get inside, somebody's going to see you.' But in actual fact we have the last house in a dead-end street and so nobody ever comes by. I went up to Steve and said, 'You care more about this goddamned car than you do about me.' He said, 'It cost us a whole lot of money. I have to take care of it, right?' And I said, 'I'm going to cost you a whole lot more if you don't take care of me.' He tried to go on washing the car but I picked up the bucket and emptied it all over his jeans. Then I unbuckled his belt and pulled his jeans halfway down his thighs. He tried to resist me but he couldn't. I was naked and wet and I don't think any man could have resisted me then. I picked up the garden hose and sprayed it all over his dick. Then I took his dick into my mouth and sucked it, while I played the hose all around his balls and all around his asshole.

"He opened the back door of the car and picked me up and lifted me into it. I don't know who wanted to fuck more urgently—him or me. I opened my legs wide and pinched each of my cunt lips between finger and thumb and stretched them apart, so that he could see right up inside me. We were both wet but that didn't matter. It made it all the more exciting. He took hold of his dick in his hand and rubbed it up and down against my cunt lips. Pale pink cunt lips and dark purple dick, and both of them shining with juice. I watched his dick disappearing into my cunt, inch by inch. In fact I stretched my lips even wider apart and lifted my head so that I could watch it sink into me. And it went all the way in, right up to his pubic hair, so that you couldn't tell which was my pubic hair and which was his.

"He fucked me better than he'd ever fucked me before. He took his dick right out of my cunt, and hesitated, and then he plunged it back in again, and that was great. Halfway through, I sat up and gave his dick another suck, and all I could taste was my own cunt juice, and that turned me on even more. When he climaxed, he climaxed deep inside me, and he shivered, and I knew that I'd won some kind of a battle, you know? I knew that I'd reminded him why we were together, and how sexy I really was.

"I didn't dress for the rest of the day. I sat on the couch watching television and I kept my legs apart so that he couldn't help looking at my cunt. He sat down next to me and he couldn't leave me alone. He kept touching my breasts and playing with my nipples and you would have thought that he'd never made love to a woman before. What turned him on more than anything else was when his sperm started to drip out of my cunt onto the couch. He put his finger inside me and gently stirred it around and around and it made this fantastic sticky noise.

"I didn't dress until seven o'clock when he took me out for a Mexican dinner. All the same, he couldn't keep his eyes off me and he couldn't stop touching me and caressing me. When we got home he couldn't wait to get his hands on me. I was soaking in the bathtub and he took off his clothes and climbed in beside me, and I think he would have fucked me in the water if he'd been able to get his dick in, but the water had washed all my juices away, and it was too difficult.

"When you walk around naked in front of your man, you suddenly realize what power you have, just because you're a woman. And I don't think there's any harm in using that power to improve your sex life, especially if you can improve it as much as I did mine. Steve never washes the car on Saturday mornings now, he's too busy with the naked woman who gives him the time of his life."

A tip: If you enjoy making love in the tub, add a tablespoonful of baby oil to the bathwater, and you will find that intercourse is much easier.

It takes self-confidence to walk around naked in front of your partner, especially if you're self-conscious about your figure. But whatever *you* think about your figure, remember that your partner fell in love with *you,* not with anybody else. He loves the way you look. He gets aroused when he sees you without any clothes on. Barbara, 27, a waitress from San Francisco, California, didn't like her partner, Brad, to see her naked because she thought that she was too fat. She was a plump child, and when she reached puberty she developed enormous breasts, a rounded stomach, and a very generous derriere.

"I was so lucky to find Brad. He came into the restaurant and we hit it off right away. He's an arts major, he's funny, he's intelligent, he's *thin.* I don't know what he ever saw in me but it must have been something because he asked me to spend a weekend with him in Sausalito, and the very first night that we were together he made love to me. Only the third guy in the universe to make love to me, I might add. He took me to meet all of his friends and they were okay, most of them, except that I did get the feeling from some of them that they were thinking 'Jesus, what's Brad doing with a fat lump like that?' I saw photographs of his previous girlfriends, too, and they were all skinny and waif-like. You know, eat your heart out, Mia Farrow.

"I had no confidence in my appearance. I did everything I could to stop Brad from seeing me naked. I locked the bathroom door when I was taking a shower. I always wore a nightdress, and I wouldn't take if off until Brad had switched off the lights. He never hassled me, but in some ways that made it worse, because I began to think that he was happy with the way things were, and that he didn't *want* to see me naked. It was kind of a no-win situation, really. But it was all because I didn't value myself. I never stopped to think, 'Why does Brad want to go on seeing me? Why does Brad want to go on making love to me?' It never occurred to me that he might like me the way I was—that he might be turned on by forty-six-inch breasts and a thirty-two-inch waist and forty-inch hips. I never once looked in the mirror and said to myself, 'You may be fat but you have a very beautiful face, and Brad loves you.' "

Barbara read an article that I wrote recently for a woman's magazine in which I said that women should never worry about their weight when it comes to sex. Your bathroom scales don't measure your sexual appetite, or how good you are in bed. A larger woman can be just as arousing as a thin one, if not more so, and even if you think that you're twenty-eight pounds overweight, you can still be the sexiest woman that *he's* ever going to meet.

You should watch your weight for reasons of health, and because larger women may find it more difficult to be athletic in bed. But it's important that you should stop thinking that you're lacking in sexual attractiveness just because you're four sizes bigger than Cindy Crawford. There are plenty of things that you can do to arouse the man in your life, or the man that you'd like to have in your life. For instance, you shouldn't put off buying sexy underwear. A G-string looks just as erotic on a larger woman as it does on a supermodel. And if you have very big breasts, you can look sensational in a quarter-cup bra.

Barbara made up her mind that she was going to be the sexiest woman that Brad had ever met. She said, "He obviously liked me for myself. My personality, what I looked like, everything. But I felt that if he was prepared to accept me physically for what I was, then I should go that extra mile and give him something in return."

Barbara's sexual generosity paid off because Brad found her startlingly sexy, so she no longer had to feel that he was doing her a favor by going out with her. Although she was not thin, her sexual techniques had Brad coming back for more, again and again. And the happier she felt about her sexual relationship, the less she ate, and the trimmer she became, so that by the time she and Brad had been going out together for seven-and-a-half months, which is when I interviewed her, she had lost over thirty-one pounds. She looked terrific, and I had to congratulate her, because she had done it not by dieting but by concentrating on her sexual happiness, and Brad's too.

"I realized that I was in competition with girls much thinner than me and much more conventionally pretty than me. So I thought to myself: I'll give him everything that a girl can give a man. I'll be wild, and uninhibited, and I'll do things that he never even dreamed of.

"I bought myself some really pretty thongs. Actually I looked better in a thong than I did in regular panties because at least they didn't make me look as if I had four behinds! I also bought myself some of the lightest, wispiest bras that I could find in my size. They didn't support me as much, but they looked so much sexier than the long-line bras that I usually wore.

"I had my hair highlighted with blonde streaks, and cut much softer. I always used to pull my hair back off my face before, but this looked much more feminine. Then I went to the cosmetics department in my local store and had my face made over. The beautician really emphasized my eyes so that they didn't look little and piggy, which is what happens when I put on too much weight.

"I fixed my nails, too. They weren't very long because I used to bite them when I was unhappy, but I trimmed them and varnished them. I don't have to wax my legs because I'm not a very hairy person, but after what I read in your book I shaved off my pubic hair and used a depilatory cream to make my pussy totally smooth.

"I met Brad after work that evening and he did a double-take when he saw me. He said, 'What's happened to *you*?' and I said, 'You.' We went for an Italian meal in this little restaurant close to Brad's office and I could tell that he liked the way I looked. Afterward we went back to my apartment and Brad opened a bottle of sparkling wine. He said, 'I want to tell you, you're the most genuine girl I ever met.' I said, 'What about the sexiest?' He kissed me and unbuttoned the front of my dress. He liked the bra.

It was the first see-through bra that he'd ever seen me wearing, and the first bra that was actually made of thin material so that he could fondle my nipples through it.

"He unbuttoned my dress all the way down and took it off. I don't think he'd ever expected to see me wearing a thong, but he liked that, too—especially since it was so small that you could see that I didn't have any pubic hair. I kissed him and took off his shirt. He plays a lot of tennis and so his body's quite fit and muscular. I took off my bra and held my bare breasts in both hands and rubbed them against his chest. Then I opened his pants and took out his cock. It was beautiful and hard and it smelled of cock, which I adore. I like a man to smell like a man. If he comes to bed smelling of nothing but soap and Calvin Klein, well, that's okay, but it's not nearly so sexy. He wanted to make love to me right there and then, but I wouldn't let him. I knelt down between his legs and held his cock in my hand. Then I took a mouthful of sparkling wine and dribbled it all over his cock and his balls, while I slowly masturbated him up and down. I took his cock into my mouth and sucked him and licked him all the way down. Then I sucked each of his balls, one after the other. When his cock was all wet and slippery I sat up and took it between my breasts. The head of it just peeped out from my cleavage and I bent my head down and licked it with the tip of my tongue.

"That's one thing I learned—when you have a

man's cock in your mouth, you're in charge. He'll do just about anything you want him to do! I can't honestly say that I liked it very much when I first did it. I was very nervous and I think I was too quick. But if you take your time and relish it—if you try licking around and around and exploring the shape of it—I think it can get quite addictive. I'd rather suck Brad's cock than suck a Nikki Bar . . . and it has a lot less calories!

"I tugged his pants the rest of the way off, and then I said, 'Come into the bedroom, I've got a surprise for you.' I don't think he could quite believe that this was happening, because I'd never been so forward with him before. I opened the drawer beside my bed and took out a jar of strawberry-scented lubricant. I knelt on the bed with my head down against the pillow. I pulled my thong out of my bottom, and then I took a handful of lubricant and smeared it all around my anus.

"Brad didn't need to be told what to do, believe me! He knelt behind me and he used his fingers to rub the lubricant around and around. That felt sensational, I never wanted it to stop. Then he pushed one finger into my anus to make sure that it was good and lubricated inside. The next thing I knew I could feel the big hard head of his cock up against my anus, pushing to get in. I did the wrong thing at first, and squeezed my anus tight. But then I pushed against him, and he slowly managed to push his cock into my bottom, inch by inch.

"For a split-second it really hurt, but then I relaxed, and I felt my insides opening out to welcome him in. He pushed himself into me so deep that I could feel his balls bumping against my bare pussy. He fucked me very slowly, reaching around to cup my breasts in his hands and massage my nipples. I could feel an orgasm coming, but it wasn't like any orgasm that I'd ever had before. It made my insides quiver. I felt so sensitive that I couldn't stand to have Brad's cock sliding in and out of my anus any longer, yet I couldn't bear for him to stop. I put one hand between my legs and I could feel his slippery cock and his balls covered in lubricant, and I was amazed to feel my anus, how wide it was stretched. My pussy was filled with juice, and I couldn't stop myself from fingering it, and then from rubbing my clitoris.

"Brad lifted my bottom higher and almost stood up on the bed behind me, his knees slightly bent, so that he could force himself into me harder and harder. He suddenly clutched my hips and climaxed. I couldn't feel his cum inside me, but it was enough to imagine it, and I had an orgasm, too. I fell sideways and I literally doubled up because I was having such spasms. Brad and I lay in each other's arms for a long time afterward, and he very gently touched and stroked my anus. He said, 'Where did you learn to do that?' and I said, 'Here, tonight. My ass was a virgin ass until now.'

"He held me very tight and I knew then that he wasn't going to let me go for a very long time."

It takes confidence and courage to initiate new sexual acts in your relationships. Barbara admitted that she was "extremely nervous" about what she was going to do that evening, and she almost didn't go through with it. But Brad's response to her oral sex was so positive that she decided to give it a try, and as it turned out, the result was highly arousing and very satisfying for both of them. Barbara says now that she and Brad have anal sex regularly and that she in now capable of taking his penis into her back passage as easily as taking it into her vagina.

I am asked a great many questions about anal sex, particularly by women who are keen to try it but don't know how to initiate it. One of the simplest ways is to take your lover's penis out of your vagina during intercourse and move it backward until his glans is pressing against your anus. If he doesn't get the message when you do this, you can then whisper, "Why don't we try it this way?"

To begin with, you may find it difficult to take your lover's penis into your anus, especially if you're feeling tense. The first few times you do it, you may also find that it hurts, depending on how well-lubricated your anus is and how forcefully your lover enters you. You may also find that certain angles of penetration are uncomfortable. Don't hesitate to tell your lover immediately if he is causing you any pain, and don't feel obliged to carry on with anal intercourse if you're not enjoying it. Some days you may feel like having his whole erection up inside you, while on other occasions you may not want even a single finger. The choice is entirely yours. Maria, 27, from Dallas, Texas, said, "I have to be wildly turned on before I can even think about anal sex. Then I adore it. But don't try it on me when I'm just having a regular roll in the hay, because then I don't enjoy it at all."

Marthe, on the other hand, a very lithe 24-year-old dancer and photographic model I met in Stockholm, Sweden, was capable of taking two fully erect penises into her anus at once. "I love it when you have two men jostling their cocks together in your ass. They fight each other and you feel like you're being completely ravaged."

If you're thinking of anal sex with a partner whose sexual history you're not 100 percent sure of, then insist that he *always* wear an extra-thick condom. Minor tears in the rectum are not uncommon during anal intercourse and the HIV virus can easily be transmitted into the bloodstream. Even couples who know that they are sexually safe use condoms during anal intercourse since the rectum is a breeding ground for virulent bacteria and there is a small risk that the man may contract an infection through his penis.

All precautions aside, anal sex can give you some extraordinary orgasmic sensations, and most men find it extremely exciting. As Tuppy Owens said,

"Once opened up, the anus is so sensitive that the right touch sends your entire body on its way to another planet. 'Feeling gorgeously full' is a million miles away from doing it justice."

Once you have learned to take your lover's penis easily into your anus, you can use your rectum as an alternative to your vagina. This enables many women to continue having intercourse during their monthly period, at a time when their sex drive is much higher than usual.

However, there is an increasing trend for couples to ignore a woman's period and go on having vaginal intercourse regardless of menstrual bleeding. Sex writer Emma Harris said, "When I'm having my period, I'm in the mood, and I don't want to waste that horny feeling. This is where my present lover comes in. He's not in the least bit worried about finding strings to tampons or getting his cock smothered in blood. Having a period is perfectly natural, and it also makes me feel more feminine and womanly. It's a sign of fertility, of womanhood, and sharing that with someone is about as intimate as you can get."

If your partner isn't squeamish about blood, lovemaking during your period can be an intensely erotic and different experience. Apart from being arousing, men find that it demystifies menstruation and makes them much more understanding about the female body and the monthly cycle. Instead of being made to stay "off limits," men become part of the experience. I have discussed menstrual sex with many different men and some of them actually look forward to "that time of the month" because of the pleasures their partners can give them when they're bleeding.

"I never would have dreamed of doing it," said 28-year-old Kathy, an auto rental manager from St. Paul, Minnesota. "But one evening I went to a company party and met Jake, who was a very good-looking guy. He took me back to my apartment and we drank some more wine and we were getting very hot and heavy, but I had to tell him that I couldn't make love to him because it was the wrong time of the month. He said he didn't care at all. He said, 'If we don't do this now, maybe we'll never have the chance again, ever.' He carried me into the bedroom and undressed me, and then undressed himself. He had a great body with a gorgeous hairy chest, and he was a wonderful kisser. He made my mouth tingle. When he started to take off my panties I was going to say no, but then I thought, If *he* doesn't mind, why should I? He put on a condom but he didn't rush me into having intercourse. He kissed and stroked my breasts and he worked his way down to my pussy very gradually. He stroked the lips of my pussy and then he opened them a little way, with two fingers, and he slipped them inside to find the string of my tampon. He tugged it out and wrapped it in tissue and dropped it beside the bed. Then he lay beside me, kissing me, and gently flicking my clitoris.

"I always feel much more responsive when I'm

having my period. A man only has to breathe on my nipples and they stick up, and my breasts always feel incredibly sensitive. Jake kept on flicking my clitoris until I began to feel that if I didn't have him inside me I was going to burst. He lifted my leg and pushed his cock into my pussy from the side, so that he could continue flicking my clitoris while he fucked me.

"I forgot that I was having a period. All I knew was that I was someplace in heaven. Jake's cock felt gigantic, and the way he pushed it into me—and hesitated—and then took it almost all the way out of me—and hesitated—that blew me away. At the same time he kept on stroking my clitoris and running his fingers all around my pussy lips.

"I was beginning to feel pretty wet, and when I lifted my head and looked down I saw that I was bleeding everywhere. There were red handprints all over my thighs and my stomach, and Jake's cock was streaked in red. I said, 'Oh God,' or something like that, but Jake kissed me and said, 'Don't you worry, you're fantastic,' and carried on fucking me.

"That's when I decided to let myself go, and enjoy every second of it. I reached down and massaged his balls and they were all slippery with blood. We twined our fingers together and stroked his cock and my pussy. Then I held my pussy open for him so that he could push himself deeper. My pussy lips were swollen because I was so turned on, and they looked as if they had been painted bright red.

"I had the kind of orgasm you only get once in a lifetime. Everything went dark. When it was all over we lay on the bed and we were both covered in blood. You should have seen the sheets, too! But I felt wonderful. I felt as if I'd done something important, something that was entirely to do with me and what I was, my generation. My mother would never have made love while she was having a period. She wouldn't even have *thought* about it. It was taboo in those days. But now things are different.

"We stripped the sheets off the bed, then we took a shower together, and that was an added bonus. We soaped each other all over, and I rubbed Jake's cock until he got hard again. He couldn't manage another climax, but that didn't matter. We held each other in the shower with the water pouring over us and it was pure magic."

The idea of menstrual sex may still shock many women who were brought up to think of periods as a "woman's problem" that shouldn't be openly discussed. But the reality is that most young men these days have been co-educated and regard menstruation as perfectly natural and not at all off-putting. With so many advertisements in the media for tampons and panty shields, "that awkward time of the month" can hardly be considered any longer to be a cause for major embarrassment.

Some sex researchers say that continuing intercourse throughout your period can help to alleviate menstrual cramps, and although I have no statistical evidence to support this claim, 31-year-old Tara from Newark, New Jersey, told me that whenever she had cramps she asked her boyfriend, Robert, to make love to her. "If you can manage to have an orgasm, that gets rid of your cramps completely."

Sometimes it seems as if the orgasm is the cure for almost any ailment, since I have had several letters from women claiming that they could clear their sinus problems by having an orgasm. Several men, too, have reported that the quickest way of clearing blocked sinuses is not to use a nasal spray but to make love.

Emma Harris is even enthusiastic about her lover giving her oral sex during her period, calling it "rainbow kisses." She says, "I feel physically closer to my lover when he's got his head between my legs and comes up for air with a red moustache. He claims it tastes pretty good, too, and enjoys the intimacy of licking me clean, gulping down my life-blood, taking a little more of me inside of him each time."

Ultimately, the secret of really great sex is to give yourself permission to enjoy any sexual pleasure that takes your fancy, and encourage your lover to give it to you. That's what I mean by taking control of your love life: ridding yourself of your hang-ups and your inhibitions, and then teaching your partner to take you wherever your sexual fancy wants to go. Carla, a 22-year-old cocktail waitress in Los Angeles, California, had a disastrous relationship with a would-be actor she met when she first arrived from

Tampa, Florida. "He was nothing but a bundle of insecurity. He used to blame me every time he failed to get a screen test. He used to blame me if his apartment was untidy or his dog was sick or if he was given a ticket for speeding. Everything was my fault. If he got drunk and couldn't get an erection that was my fault, too. In the end he started to hit me, so I packed my bags and I walked out.

"I was real lonesome for two or three months, but I was determined that I was going to stay in Los Angeles and make myself a career as a dancer. But then I met Rick and his brother Dave and their friend Lenny. They'd all been at school together . . . they were like the Three Musketeers, you know. They worked for this car wash, but that was just their daytime job. What they really lived for was a rock group they were trying to get together. They were sure that they were going to be rich and famous. I heard them a couple of times. They were terrible. But they were great guys. They were so good looking, all of them. Rick and his brother had brown curly hair and the bluest eyes. Rick looked like Jim Morrison before he got fat. Lenny was blond and shy and always reminded me of River Phoenix.

"I met them when I took my car to be cleaned. They must have liked the look of me because they invited me to a party they were going to that night. I said, 'sure.' I mean, this was the first time that anybody had invited me out since I walked out on Calvin. I dressed up that night in my shortest, sexiest, purple satin dress and no underwear and I told myself that I was going to be the sexiest woman in the whole place.

"It isn't easy to do that, to make yourself feel confident and sexy, especially when you've been living with a guy like Calvin who's always bringing you down and making you feel that everything is your fault, no matter what. He was drunk once, when he was driving, and he hit the curb. That was my fault, too, because I'd been talking at the time, and I'd distracted him. It was misery. It really was. And I still wonder how many women have to go through misery like that every single day, because they're living with guys like Calvin, and they're too insecure to leave them.

"Calvin never made me feel sexy or pretty or anything. If I wore a low-cut dress he used to go crazy, saying that I was a whore and a bitch and I was trying to make him look like a fool in front of his friends. The only reason I had the confidence to go out with Rick and Dave and Lenny was because I read your book [*Secrets of the Sexually Irresistible Woman*] and you said that every woman is sexually attractive if she believes that she is; and you made me believe.

"The party was wild. There was a Mexican band and crowds of people and mountains of tortillas and empenadas and burritos. Rick, Dave, and Lenny took care of me all the time. They danced with me, they made sure that my glass was always full, they brought me burritos in the palms of their hands. I felt so sexy that night, I can't tell you. I felt sexy because I didn't have any inhibitions, I didn't mind what I did, and I didn't mind who I did it with. That feeling is so liberating, you know? That understanding that sex doesn't *hurt* anybody, it makes them feel good. I stood on the table and I danced, and everybody was clapping and cheering. I flipped up my dress so that everybody could see that I wasn't wearing any panties, and the applause was amazing. Maybe I was just a little drunk, but more than that I was confident and happy. So a hundred people were looking at my cunt? I'm glad they liked it. I'm glad they wanted to look. I flipped my dress up at the back, too, and showed them my tushy.

"I don't know how long the party went on . . . maybe til three or four. Then the guys drove me back to their house in Coldwater Canyon. It wasn't much of a place, kind of a bachelor's shack. But it was pretty neat and tidy, with Indian blankets on the floors. Rick lit a fire because it was getting cold and Dave opened a bottle of wine and the three of them sat around and strummed their guitars and played me some of their songs.

"I leaned up against Rick and he kissed me. I sat up a little and kissed him back. That night I felt that I could have whatever I wanted. Rick put down his guitar and slipped my dress up over my head, so that I was completely naked except for my shoes. He started to unbutton his shirt, and while he did, Dave came over and kissed me, too; and then Lenny came up behind him and felt my breasts. He had a way of pulling my nipples and rolling them between his fingers that was so sexy.

"Rick was naked now, and Dave started to undress, too. We hardly said a word between us. I don't think we had to. Like, a situation like that doesn't need any explanations, does it? Or justifications, or anything. I was a young woman who felt like making love to three young men, and that was all there was to it. Nothing harmful, nothing dangerous, nothing adulterous. It was sex, pure and simple, and it was really great sex.

"I lay down on the Navajo rug in front of the fire, and all three of them were all over me. Three stiff cocks, it was fantastic! I took Rick's cock in one hand and Lenny's in the other and gave them a good hard rubbing. Then Dave knelt down, right over my face, so that I could suck his balls and lick his cock. It was amazing how different their cocks were. Rick's was thick and heavy, with veins that stuck out. Dave's was smoother and longer. Lenny's curved upward, with a bright pink wedge-shaped head on it.

"I sucked all three of them, one after the other, and then I tried to suck all three of them at once, but they were much too big to get into my mouth! At the same time they were stroking me and touching me and licking me. Rick and Dave both went down on me together, with Dave holding my cunt open while Dave licked it, and then both of them licking, two tongues licking my cunt simultaneously, while I licked Lenny's bright pink cock and played with his balls.

"Rick brought out some condoms and they all rolled one on. It was great to watch them. In fact I rolled Rick's condom on for him. Dave lay on his back on the rug and Rick helped me to climb on top of him. Rick took hold of Dave's cock and guided it into my cunt. You don't know how good that felt, when that slid into me. It wasn't like Calvin's cock at all. It was long and hard and it seemed to poke into parts of me that Calvin had never been able to reach. Mind you, Calvin had never let me sit on top of him. He thought it was unmanly, or something.

"While Dave was fucking me, Rick and Lenny were touching me everywhere, touching my breasts, stroking my thighs, tickling the soles of my feet, touching my cunt, fingering my asshole. It was out of this world. I could see us in the dressing-table mirror on the other side of the bedroom. Rick knelt behind me and I felt him rubbing something greasy around my asshole. I didn't realize it at the time, but it was Hollywood Margarine. Lenny took hold of my bottom and spread it wide, and then I felt Rick's cock up against my asshole. I thought, 'Oh, no . . . I'm going to be fucked by two men at once.' But then I thought, 'Yes, I want it. I really want it,' and I opened myself up so that Rick could push his cock right up into my ass. The feeling was out of this world. I was so excited that I started to scream and jump up and down even faster. I wanted more and more and more! I wished I had three holes so that I could take all of them in.

"But Lenny was rubbing margarine on Rick's ass now. I could see him in the mirror. He crouched behind Rick and he pushed his cock into Rick's anus. I could feel Rick's cock swelling even bigger, and he started to fuck my ass even harder. I put my hands down behind me and I felt three pairs of balls, all greasy with margarine and slippery with juice. I fondled all of them, and Dave started to groan because he was getting close to his climax and didn't want to come so soon.

"He couldn't hold it back any longer, and I kissed him while he filled his condom up with sperm. Then Rick climaxed, and Lenny did, too, and the two of them fell sideways on the bed panting and laughing. I took off their condoms for them, and masturbated each of them for a while, until the sperm on their cocks dried.

"About an hour later, we did it again, but this time Rick was underneath and Lenny went into my ass and Dave went into *him*. It was the most extreme sex I've ever been involved in, but there was so much laughter and affection that I couldn't think of it as wrong or perverted or anything like that. I asked the boys afterward if they were gay or bisexual, but they said that they weren't. They made love to each other because they enjoyed it and it was a way for all three of them to make love to one girl simultaneously.

"To start with, the boys were in control because I'd never gotten involved in anything like that before. It was exciting at first because it was such a forbidden thing to do, but after I'd been seeing them for about two weeks I began to feel very unsatisfied because they always climaxed so quickly and I never managed to reach an orgasm. I also felt that they were having sex with me just to please themselves and they weren't particularly worried about what it was like for me.

"That's when *I* took control. Before I let them have intercourse with me, I made each of them go down on me in turn, and lick my cunt until I had an orgasm . . . all three of them, so I always had three orgasms before we'd even started. I didn't just lie there while they went down on me. I sucked their cocks and masturbated them . . . it's great trying to get two cocks into your mouth at once . . . and I did other things, too, like stroking their balls and sticking my finger up their asses. After that I let them make love to me, and it was always me who got to choose who was going to fuck me and which way. Sometimes I got them to have sex together while I just lay back and watched them and masturbated myself. You don't know how exciting it is to see a man's cock disappearing into another man's ass. Once or twice I sucked them while they were being fucked, and they really went for that. Other times I masturbated two of them by hand while I sucked the third one's cock.

"I guess some people would say that what I was doing was very immoral, but it wasn't like that at all. The love between us was something very special that you only find once in a lifetime. Once I was in control of what was happening, those three boys treated me like a princess, and they gave me the most satisfying lovemaking I've ever had, or ever will, unless I meet another three guys with the same free-and-easy attitude toward sex.

"I know that I'm a much better lover than I was. I don't have any inhibitions about doing anything, and most men find that amazing. I'm almost always satisfied because I can make my lovers do what I want them to do. Most of the time they don't even realize that it's me who's controlling when they make love to me, and how they do it, and how fast. But I can tell you that they always keep coming back for more!"

You don't have to have a threesome to explore different sexual positions and different sexual techniques, you can try them all out on the same man. But as we've seen, it's valuable to use your imagination give your lover a variety of sexual personalities. One day, for instance, you can expect him to treat you smoothly and gently. Another day you can coax him into treating you rough. You can control the agenda by the way you behave: you'll be surprised how responsive most men are to your differing sexual moods.

We've come a long way since we first discussed

meditation techniques at the beginning of this book. Now it's time for you to go out and discover really great sex for yourself. Always remember to never be afraid of trying something new, and that you should never allow yourself to be bullied—either physically or emotionally—into sexual acts that you really *don't* want to do. For most of us, really extreme sex is something to be tried only once or twice, or simply fantasized about, but even if you think about it and never do actually do it, it can still add spice to your love life, and it can still liberate you and make you feel more adventurous.

Promise yourself that you're going to meditate and rid yourself of your sexual inhibitions. Promise yourself you're going to take control of your love life, for your benefit and for your partner's benefit, too. Because after you've done that, the whole world of really great sex is out there, just waiting for you to enjoy it.

57 Ways to Have Really Great Sex

1: Go to a party with no panties on (but don't tell your partner until halfway through the evening).
2: Send for a mail-order sex catalog (i.e. The Xandria Collection, P.O. Box 31039, San Francisco, CA, 94131-9988; or Desires, 100 Glenn Road, Suite A-9, Sterling, VA, 20164; or any one of many more) and order any sex toy that takes your fancy. And *use* it.
3: Buy yourself some erotic underwear and wear it all day to work.
4: Spend an entire day naked, whether your partner's with you or not.
5: Masturbate yourself to orgasm before you get out of bed in the morning.
6: Masturbate your partner to orgasm before he can get out of bed in the morning.

7: Give your partner oral sex while he's asleep.
8: Give your partner oral sex while he's watching television.
9: Tell your partner your most extreme sexual fantasy.
10: Insist that your partner tells you his most extreme sexual fantasy.
11: Blindfold your partner while you're making love.
12: Masturbate your partner until he climaxes over your breasts.
13: Call your partner at work and tell him how much you want him to make love to you. Be graphic. Be very graphic!
14: Don't allow your partner to have intercourse with you until he's given you an orgasm.
15: Don't allow your partner to have vaginal intercourse with you. Insist that it has to be anal, or not at all.
16: Sit on your partner's face and give him a juicy sexual facial.
17: Suck your partner's toes, and then insert his big toe into your vagina.
18: Shave your pubic hair into the shape of a heart, or an arrow, or a star.
19: Shave off your pubic hair completely.
20: Have your birth sign tattooed on your behind.
21: Have your vaginal lips pierced.
22: Greet your lover in erotic underwear when he comes home from work.

23: Insist that your lover make love to you the minute he walks in the door.

24: Visit your lover at work and lift your skirt (when nobody else is looking) to show him that you've shaved your vulva.

25: Sit on your lover's erect penis and meditate, Tantric-style, not moving, and holding off your orgasm for as long as possible.

26: Shave off your lover's pubic hair so that his penis and his testicles are completely bald. Then give him the licking of his life!

27: Play with your lover's nipples in the same way that you like yours to be played with.

28: Give your lover oral sex and swallow his semen.

29: Invite your partner to watch you urinating. Let him touch you if he wants to.

30: Hold your partner's penis while he urinates. If it's outdoors, and it's snowing, you can draw an arrow-pierced heart to show him how much you love him.

31: Pour maple syrup over your vulva and invite him to lick it off.

32: Insert a peeled banana into your vagina and see if he can eat it all.

33: Smother his penis with your favorite ice-cream and make sure that you clean it off completely. Rocky Road is especially good!

34: Take him aside at a social function and get your hand into his pants. Make sure he has trouble doing them up again.

35: When he comes home from work, greet him at the door wearing nothing but garter belt, stockings, and stiletto heels.
36: Buy the sleaziest, sexiest underwear you can find (crotchless panties, open-fronted cat suits) and wear it to bed.
37: Invite him to make love to you outside . . . preferably someplace where there's a high risk of discovery, such as a downtown alley or a public park.
38: Wet your finger and insert it into his anus while he's asleep, then gently jiggle his cock to wake him up.
39: See how wide apart you can stretch your legs during intercourse. If you're very athletic, you may even be able to wrap your feet behind your head.
40: Ask him to wear your dirty panties to work, underneath his suit.
41: Call him at work and tell him about all of those sexual fantasies that you didn't dare to tell him to his face.
42: Flavor your anus with strawberry or cinnamon or mint and invite him to lick it for you.
43: Buy or rent a selection of pornographic videos and ask him to watch them with you.
44: Ask him for intercourse at unexpected times of the day: just after breakfast, or halfway through the afternoon, or the minute you come back from the market.

45: Wake him up in the middle of the night and demand sex.

46: Buy him some leather bondage gear—penis restraints and straps and masks and demand that he behave like a slave.

47: Tell him to spank you every time you misbehave.

48: Wear garter belt and stockings and *shoes* to bed.

49: Do your aerobic exercises together—in the nude.

50: Show him how you masturbate, but don't let him touch you while you're doing it. He's there to learn!

51: Go jogging together, some place remote, in the nude.

52: Make love in the open air in the rain.

53: Leave an erotic e-mail on his laptop.

54: Set up a video camera and perform a striptease . . . then invite him to join you in bed while you watch it.

55: Videotape your lovemaking, and then make love while your tape is playing.

56: Spend half an hour in silence, touching and caressing his naked body without making love.

57: Think of the most extreme sex act you can, and then dare to try it.

Above all, have a really great time!